THE EMOTIONAL TRUTH OF DREAMS

This book explores what we can learn from dreams, both nocturnal and waking, through their revelations of emotional truths, and how these truths can inform psychotherapeutic practice, spiritual practice, and everyday life.

The co-authors—both psychotherapists and artists—demonstrate the path of awakening not only *from* dreams but also *to* and *through* dreams. They suggest that to dream is to realize grace. Further, they apprentice grace by developing and deepening relationship to the soul's divine gifts and receiving the wondrous offerings of vivid dreamlife. Through contemplation of more than 13 dreams, the authors share their collaborative dream dialogues and reflections. In this process, new meanings, questions, and revelations about the life of the soul emerge. They show how to cultivate the practice of deeply listening to our dreams and the emotional truths they harbor by growing awareness and receptivity to our psyche's enigmatic expressions.

With rich dream dialogues and a focus on learning from dreams together, this book is essential reading for psychoanalysts, psychotherapists, and anyone wanting to explore how dreams can help us better understand ourselves in relationship to the mystery of the soul, to each other, and to the world.

emotionaltruthofdreams.com

Willow Pearson Trimbach, PsyD, LMFT, MT-BC, is Professor and Director of Clinical Training, Clinical Psychology Department, California Institute of Integral Studies. Dr. Pearson Trimbach practices psychotherapy in the Bay Area, California, where she sees adults and provides consultation and supervision. She is a psychologist, psychotherapist, music therapist, author, singer, and songwriter.

Eva Tuschman Leonard, LMFT, is a psychotherapist, writer, and visual artist residing in Northern California. Her first book, *Bodywork*, is a meditation on illness, grief, and desire told through her drawings and written reflections.

Psyche and Soul: Psychoanalysis, Spirituality and Religion in Dialogue Book Series

Series Editors: Jill Salberg and Melanie Suchet

The *Psyche and Soul: Psychoanalysis, Spirituality and Religion in Dialogue* series explores the intersection of psychoanalysis, spirituality and religion. By promoting dialogue, this series provides a platform for the vast and expanding interconnections, mutual influences, and points of divergence amongst these disciplines. Extending beyond western religions of Judaism, Christianity and Islam, the series includes Eastern religions, contemplative studies, mysticism, and philosophy. By bridging gaps, opening the vistas, and responding to increasing societal yearnings for more spirituality in psychoanalysis, *Psyche and Soul* aims to cross these disciplines, fostering a more fluid interpenetration of ideas.

For a full list of titles in this series, please visit the Routledge website: https://www.routledge.com/Psyche-and-Soul/book-series/PSYSOUL

'This is an intimate book—intuitive, illuminating, and inspiring. Willow Pearson Trimbach and Eva Tuschman Leonard's engaged, relational exploration of waking dreams and nighttime dreams in psyche time opens the reader to multiple dimensions of what Bion called emotional truth. Through their dream dialogues, touching longings, realizations, losses, and creative expressions, dreams are held as guides from the mystery of the soul. The offering of these dream dialogues invites you to partner your own dreamlife, as a lifelong path of contact with the depths. Listening for grace is an expressed method of their dream practice, helping the reader to gain psychotherapeutic and spiritual access that honors and opens resonant sources yet unknown. This is a wonderful further exploration into our human experience as feeling and dreaming beings.'

Michael Eigen, *author of* The Challenge of Being Human, The Psychoanalytic Mystic, Psychic Deadness, *and* The Sensitive Self

'This book is a genuinely artistic and inspiring masterpiece—deeply enriching and exceptionally well-written. Chapter by chapter, the authors guide us with creative vision and insight toward the emotional truths of dreams. By inviting the reader into their intimate conversations, they allow qualities of aliveness to emerge, and we are changed by it—both personally and professionally. This captivating work illuminates psychoanalytic and psychotherapeutic thinking with brilliance, making it essential reading for anyone interested in exploring dreams as a path to self-inquiry. It also shows how, through engaging with dream dialogues, we come to nest ourselves—and others—more deeply.'

Jani Santamaría Linares, *PhD, editor of* Bion, Dreamwork and the Oneiric Dimensions of the Mind *and co-editor of The Bion Seminars at the A-Santamaría Association*

'Willow and Eva have crafted an insightful, heartfelt, and truly original book that is sure to delight any explorer of the nocturnal mind. Ever since Plato, the power of dialogue has been engaged for transformation. This elegant book is about authentic dialogue—with our deeper self, with each other, and with reality. Rigorous, reflective, and infinitely wise, these gifted guides will take you to the treasures that await you within and show you to share that wealth with the world.'

Andrew Holecek, *author of* Dream Yoga

'Through this book, Willow Pearson Trimbach and Eva Tuschman Leonard carve an astonishing new path of dialogue with multiple intuitive perspectives demonstrating their scholarly care and freedom. Dreamwork in this context is the awakening of the dreamer to liberatory emotional truths. They push the insistence on interpretation of dream to a radical turn—a new method of engaged dream practice, arguing for an ecological interconnectedness extending from the hollow of the dream navel to the ever-evolving Anima Mundi. An unanticipated outcome of this work is its silent reparative impulse to heal the history of psychoanalysis by bringing Freudian,

Jungian, and mystical traditions closer in "withness" to a common concern—for life, death, or what dreams may come.'

Shifa Haq, *assistant professor, Ambedkar University Delhi, author of* In Search of Return: Mourning the Disappearances in Kashmir

'With this compelling new book, Willow Pearson Trimbach and Eva Tuschman Leonard invite you to awaken to the deep mystery of dreaming—at once a dialogical practice embracing the fullness of our being, as well as a path toward the more we have yet to become. Accepting their invitation to "sing your dreams" might just open your soul to growth, grace, and love you didn't know were waiting for you.'

Robin Bagai, *PsyD, lecturer and editor of* A Michael Eigen Companion: Moments of Wisdom from a Psychoanalytic Mystic

'In this deeply touching dialogical work, Willow Pearson Trimbach and Eva Tuschman Leonard re-vision the interpersonal as incubator to our oneiric dimension of being. For these authors, dreams as nested ontology give birth to a *third body* able to nourish our communal dream-weaving capacities—the psychic tissue needed to "hear" our perennial pre-caesurian and caesurian murmurations, screams, and vanishing points. Read Willow Pearson Trimbach and Eva Tuschman Leonard and welcome your re-"living," your silent rebirths, and nourish your ordinary waking perception of reality.'

Loray Daws, *PhD, DPsa, psychoanalyst and clinical psychologist, author of* Introduction to the Work of Michael Eigen

'Luminous and oneiric, *The Emotional Truth of Dreams* returns dreaming to the heart of psychoanalysis. This book reads like a dream—porous, shimmering, unhurried—its pages opening emotional truth across space and time. With exceptional grace, Willow Pearson Trimbach and Eva Tuschman Leonard sing the dream that awakens and expands the heart-mind. Sublime and enlarging, dreams in these pages represent, connect, and transform.'

Shalini Masih, *author of* Psychoanalytic Conversations with States of Spirit Possession: Beauty in Brokenness

'In an era of doom-scrolling social media feeds in order to instantly receive overwhelming artificial information from people we probably won't ever meet, Willow Pearson Trimbach and Eva Tuschman Leonard offer us a calming, nourishing alternative: to attentively get to know ourselves through intimate psychic dialogue with another human being via the timeless wisdom of dreams. It was a transformative pleasure to accompany them on the co-reverie landscape of their elegant soul-touching text, and discover alongside their generous first-person-voices, the worlds of irreplaceable healing, connection, and understanding that open when we make time for dreaming together.'

Adam Shechter, *LCSW, author of* The Phantasy of the Socialist Heart and The Uroboros, Free Associations

THE EMOTIONAL TRUTH OF DREAMS

Learning from Dream Dialogues in Psychotherapeutic and Spiritual Practice

Willow Pearson Trimbach
and Eva Tuschman Leonard

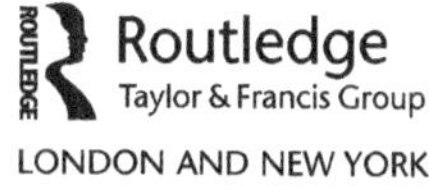

LONDON AND NEW YORK

First published 2026
by Routledge
4 Park Square, Milton Park, Abingdon, Oxon OX14 4RN

and by Routledge
605 Third Avenue, New York, NY 10158

Routledge is an imprint of the Taylor & Francis Group, an informa business

British Library Cataloguing-in-Publication Data
A catalogue record for this book is available from the British Library

ISBN: 978-1-032-97042-4 (hbk)
ISBN: 978-1-032-96470-6 (pbk)
ISBN: 978-1-003-59186-3 (ebk)

DOI: 10.4324/9781003591863

Typeset in Times New Roman
by KnowledgeWorks Global Ltd.

www.emotionaltruthofdreams.com

To Chinnamunda/Chinnamasta, Simhamukha, and Yum Chenmo, none other than Cunda Tara, Saraswati, and Mary revealed, for oracular blessings of wrathful and peaceful compassion and for showing the way.

To Mahamayuri, queen peahen bodhisattva of the (past/present) future, for Dreaming This.

To Grace herself, in all her infinite variety.

Willow Pearson Trimbach

For my mother, Jana Silverman Tuschman, who explored the path of feminine wisdom ahead of me so that I, too, could learn to listen to and trust my own intuition. Her incredible creativity has enriched my life beyond measure.

Eva Tuschman Leonard

CONTENTS

FOREWORD

Through their intimate dialogues, Willow Pearson Trimbach and Eva Tuschman Leonard offer us a rare glimpse into how human beings can connect with the living, breathing world of dreams. Eva and Willow explore dreams as two soul friends who are psychotherapists and artists with deep, committed spiritual practices. Willow, a musician, singer, and music therapist, and Eva, a visual artist and ceramicist, connected in 2014, and their paths converged around their shared personal and professional interests. Their conversations morphed from "How are you?" to "How is your dream life?" I like to imagine the kind of world we all may live in if this were considered part of normal human discourse.

Together, Eva and Willow wove the tapestry of this book's dream passages, both nighttime and waking. By allowing us into their private conversations, we enter with them into their process of dream incubation. They walk us through their process of reflection, dreaming, recording their dreams, and revisiting them together over months or years. We witness their mutual tending, seeing how their dreams deepen, unfold in layers, and reveal unconscious dimensions. By spending an hour's focus on a single dream, shared across multiple sittings, Willow and Eva teach us how to let dream images live and breathe. The relational container between them enriched the dreambody that co-created space for their dreams to speak.

Nested Dreams

Their dialogues are *not* therapy. Yet their dialogues *are* clearly *therapeutic*. These are two friends, both therapists, who come together to show us that friendships and human relationships can literally be built on dreams! They listen with openness, vulnerability, and curiosity. This book, thereby, affirms that dreams are quintessentially human. Theory and scholarship inform, but do not define. Theory is translated into lived inquiry and embodied experience.

Generously sharing their mutual process of connecting over their dreams, Eva and Willow demonstrate how dreams are living presences, emotional truths that pulse within us and are inherently relational. They deftly show how dreams and dreamers are interrelated to each other and our inner and outer worlds, expressing the concept of *nested dreams*. Nested dreams permeate dimensions of self and other, inner and outer, experience and imagination, reality and memory.

In a kindred manner, when Willow beckoned me to write this foreword, our lunch discussion stimulated me to share one of the first dreams I brought to my analysis nearly thirty years ago:

> *I am on a train going through Italy's countryside. In another car, I hear loud voices, stomping boots, guns clicking, and gunshots firing repeatedly. I am standing in the aisle because I don't have a seat and clutching my baby doll. Suddenly, the train dramatically veers right. I stumble and land right into a man's lap, sitting in the nearest seat to my right. He is welcoming and kind. He smiles and asks my doll's name, and I reply, "Chapeau." I relax into his arms, holding my baby doll tightly.*

Consistent with nested dreams, this dream has been particularly memorable because, unbeknownst to me, it revealed truths about my past, present, and future. This dream initially provided insight into a challenging professional experience I was going through at the time, which affirmed my gut feeling about it. The dream allowed me to reflect on its impact on my life. I made hard decisions that required a significant change in my professional life.

A decade after I had this dream, I came to learn that my dream also contained layers of knowledge that exceeded the limits of what I could consciously know or understand at the time. My three-year-old daughter unknowingly and spontaneously named her first baby doll "Chapeau." Although Paris is one of my all-time favorite places, this word is from a language that my family doesn't use or speak and holds no personal meaning. Part of this dream was *precognitive*, meaning it expressed the future.

Perhaps even more uncanny, five years after my daughter named her doll "Chapeau," and fifteen years after I dreamt this dream, uncharacteristically, my Dad shared fragments of a traumatic childhood memory, something he had never before shared with me: he was on a train in Italy when Mussolini's soldiers stormed the car and shot several passengers. My Dad described a little girl, trembling in fear, clutching her baby doll.

Had I dreamt aspects of my Dad's experience that he had not shared with me? What memory was I inheriting? What field of truth had I stumbled into? In his theory of the "subliminal self," poet, philologist, psychical researcher, and founder of the Society of Psychical Research, Frederic W. H. Myers (1943), suggested that parts of our consciousness operate subliminally, beneath the ordinary threshold of awareness, and can tap into an expanded field of consciousness, including the world of intuitions and dreams. From this subliminal stratum, he proposes we can also access knowledge of events beyond our direct experience—including what we call telepathy, precognition, and retrocognition.

My dream expressed what Myers termed a *retrocognitive dream*, which reveals knowledge of past events that the dreamer could not have known, recalled, or deduced from conventional means or mental processes. My dream may have been such a retrocognitive experience. Additionally, it wove multiple threads together: a past I did not know, a future that would one day unfold, and a present moment of symbolic truth. It invited me to feel, remember, and reflect, which inspired change and growth. The dream captured the present moment as well as memory and prophecy.

Precognitive and Retrocognitive Dreams: Theory and Scholarship

Through theories about consciousness and dreams, depth psychologists and psychoanalysts can help us understand precognitive and retrocognitive dreams. Psychoanalytic thinkers have long explored how the past shapes the psyche, not only through biographical experience but also through the unconscious transmission of affects, patterns, experiences, and meaning. Simultaneously, psychoanalysis also emphasizes the continual growth of the personality and its influence on our future development.

Retrocognitive and precognitive dreams—those involving apparent knowledge of the past or anticipation of the future speak to both our past and future. Mainstream psychology and science are often skeptical of these dreams, citing inconclusive research findings, and attributing them to factors such as forgotten memories, cryptomnesia, coincidence, psychopathology, the "Barnum effect," and suggestibility. Yet, a growing body of research and theory has explored their psychological dimensions and possible explanatory mechanisms.

Empirical studies have confirmed that reports of precognitive dreams are relatively common, with approximately 15–30 percent of individuals reporting at least one such experience (Mossbridge et al., 2014). Valášek et al. (2014) found no correlation between precognitive dreaming and general psychopathology. Instead, they are associated with specific personality traits, including *absorption*—the capacity to become deeply immersed in internal experiences—and *transliminality*, a tendency toward heightened sensitivity to internal and external stimuli. Additionally, psychological variables, such as individuals with higher dream-recall frequency and more positive attitudes toward dreams, report more precognitive dream experiences (Schredl, 2009; Thalbourne & Houran, 2000; Valášek et al., 2014). Individuals who score higher on measures of intuition, fantasy proneness, and openness to spiritual or mystical experiences are also more likely to report these dreams (Krippner & Friedman, 2010).

Some of the earliest controlled experimental work in the area of dream telepathy was conducted at Maimonides Medical Center by Stanley Krippner and colleagues. Under controlled laboratory conditions, they found that dreamers could access information beyond ordinary sensory channels, providing evidence for theories of non-local consciousness and dream-based psi phenomena (Krippner et al., 1971).

Such research findings can reinforce psychoanalytic dream theories, notably C. G. Jung's. Jung posited that "dreams are like windows that allow us to look in, or to listen in to that psychological process which is continually going on in our unconscious" (1988, pp. 236–237). He asserted that dreams *reveal* far more than they conceal, and their revelatory function may encompass material from our past, present, and future as well as extrasensory experiences. That is, dreams can be *telepathic* (occur through communication between minds), *clairvoyant* (occur through information transmitted independent of the senses), or *precognitive* (foretell the future) (Jung, 1964, p. 51). Jung has noted that a dream that expresses news before it reaches the dreamer in their waking life "is something that happens fairly frequently," thereby, asserting it is part of how our psyche works rather than being paranormal (1952/1969, CW 8, ¶854). Jung notes:

> Thus dreams may sometimes announce certain situations long before they actually happen. This is not necessarily a miracle … Many crises in our lives have a long unconscious history. We move toward them step by step unaware of the dangers that are accumulating. But what we consciously fail to see is frequently perceived by our unconscious, which can pass the information on through dreams.
>
> (1964, p. 36)

Similarly, psychoanalyst James Grotstein found that "the dream represents the product of an intelligence or coherence that has access to memory and hidden emotions and can construct a narrative that is capable of meaningful decipherment" (2000, p. 19). "In this respect it is a revelatory function" (1981, p. 410; quoted in Merkur, 2010, p. 258).

Jung expounded on how dreams reflect a less accessible, acausal layer of consciousness and experience that expresses intuitive, symbolic, and transpersonal dimensions of knowing, which challenge conventional notions of time and causality. Dreams serve as portals to the unconscious, including the collective unconscious—a reservoir of archetypes, ancestral imagery, and transpersonal wisdom. From this perspective, both retrocognitive and precognitive dreams may transcend literal temporality, stimulating latent material in vivid, emotionally charged images that seek to express psychic material not yet—or no longer—accessible to the conscious mind.

Retrocognitive and precognitive dreams can be viewed as symbolic expressions of psychological truths that resonate with inherited symbols, collective experience, transgenerational trauma, archetypal motifs, and the soul's relationship to time and memory, giving rise to emotionally charged images that feel ancient yet intimately personal. Similarly, they may illustrate Jung's idea of the "prospective function" of dreams by illuminating emerging patterns in psychological development before they are consciously recognized.

Jung's concept of the *psychoid*, which describes a realm that bridges the psychic and somatic and works through processes that may not be reducible to either the physical or the psychological (Jung, 1954/1960), provides additional insight. The psychoid represents the interconnection between psyche and matter, reflecting the interplay and lack of differentiation between the psyche and the body (Jung, 1952/1969). Jung theorized that archetypes are psychoid structures—existing in a realm that connects the unconscious psyche with the somatic, collective, and transpersonal. They are not simply inherited psychological patterns that get passed along in a Lamarckian manner (Jung, 1954/1960). Symbolic and anomalous phenomena—such as telepathy, synchronicity, and precognitive or retrocognitive dreams—can emerge out of this liminal place where archetypes reside. Thus, when an individual dreams of a future or past event that they could not have consciously known, this may reflect an encounter with the psychoid level of the unconscious, where time-bound distinctions are dissolved. The dream might symbolize or even directly express events that linear cognition cannot, but are nevertheless registered or "known" in this psychoid matrix.

Precognitive dreams could be understood as symbolic or literal intrusions of information from the psychoid realm into the conscious psyche, facilitated by dream states where ego boundaries are relaxed. Likewise, retrocognitive dreams may reflect resonance with the psychoid field that holds traces of lived or collective memory (Main, 2007). Such dreams could be seen as experiential evidence of a psyche that is unconfined to present sensory knowledge or memory, one that taps into a transpersonal and acausal domain interconnecting time, matter, and being.

Jung's theory of *synchronicity*, or meaningful coincidences, is relevant here. It posits that synchronicities emerge from an underlying acausal order that expresses meaning and reflects the interconnection between psyche and matter. For example, dreaming of a future event that later comes true, is a synchronicity. Therefore, it is neither purely psychic material, but psychoid in nature—intersecting with the material world yet symbolically expressed through the dream (Jung, 1952/1969). In clinical practice, these synchronistic dreams can be met as invitations to explore the enduring mysteries of the unconscious mind and the spiritual psyche through an approach I have referred to as "synchronicity-informed psychotherapy" (Marlo, 2022).

Additionally, Wilfred Bion (1962) suggested that the mind may register emotional experiences before they are fully available to consciousness, aligning with the idea that dreams can express knowledge of previous events or anticipate future psychic states. Similarly, Marion Milner and Thomas Ogden also view dreams as temporal bridges that integrate dissociated or latent material—whether forward-looking or backward-glancing (Ogden, 2004). These ideas provide further lenses for understanding these temporally complex dreams.

A Book for Dreamers

In their introduction, Eva and Willow declare that this book is for dreamers—by which they mean every one of us. As they aspire further, the book awakens us to living dreams, by becoming attentive not only *from* dreaming but also *to* it. Eva and Willow offer a practice of liberation: a humbling, direct path available to all who listen and receive. In conversation with our dreams, we deepen our relationship with ourselves, with each other, and with the cosmos.

One common myth they center on is that dreams are not real. As this book will present and demonstrate, dreams are very real. My train dream, uncannily, expressed realities from my past, present, and future, revealing that dreams can communicate emotional truths and sometimes even literal truths. Perhaps this is why the phrase "a dream come true," they muse, has such enduring meaning. When we listen and engage deeply with our dreams, we can hear those emotional truths and sometimes encounter literal truths from our past, present, and future. Such is the mystery of dreams, which are unconstrained by logic and conventional timelines.

Willow and Eva's treatise on dreams is woven from perspectives that span relational psychoanalysis, integral theory, family systems, Bion, Jung, transpersonal psychology, spiritual practice, and artistic doing—painting, singing, ceramics—as well as lived reciprocity with animals and nature and many spiritual threads: Buddhist, Jewish, Quaker, Christian-Gnostic, Catholic, Métis-Cree, and more. This potpourri of perspectives creates a rich container that the dreambody, or third body, can inhabit. This *dreambody* is the relational soulspace formed through our attunement to dream images, one another, and deeper realms of Being.

Their book is not an academic survey of dream theory or a how-to manual. It is a lived inquiry, and through narrative examples drawn from their own dream lives, Eva and Willow reveal what they long for and discover as they engage with their dreaming selves, individually and collaboratively.

This book aspires to inspire you to engage in conversation with your dreams—no matter how you dream: nighttime, waking, artistic, mundane, or extraordinary. The shared dream dialogues contained here have been profoundly transformative for the authors. They hope that this practice of listening, reflecting, and holding dreams reverently will catalyze liberation, meaning-making, and spiritual attunement in clinicians and layreaders alike.

Living Emotional Truth: Apprenticeship to Grace

Willow and Eva affirm the value of "emotional truth" as expressed in the world of dreams. Dreams are not ephemera or fantasies but, as Bion articulated, *emotional truths*. They illustrate how emotional experiences open a gateway to emotional truth waiting beyond that door. Emotional truths are not merely feelings—it is the more profound wisdom that emerges through feeling. Emotional experience is raw material, while emotional truth is its refined essence. Like Bion's "O," emotional truth is the unknown caught within feeling. Getting there requires diving past the surface, often inaccessible, except when inhabiting the realms of dreamt mystery.

The thirteen chapters and the afterword of the book gift readers with emotional truth. Through their shared lived experience, we learn how to edge toward emotional truth, the core intelligence encrypted within each dream. It is a dream practice in which they experience being fully awake and touched by grace, which is not accidental but dependent, they entreat, on the quality of the approach. Reverent, gentle, curious attention invites in great things, including dreams that kindle exploration and growth.

Within the soul's mysterious realm, Eva and Willow show us how grace is the felt sense of sacredness. They demonstrate how we can encounter it by deepening our receptivity and allowing ourselves to be touched by something larger than ourselves.

Historically, Eva and Willow underscore that dreams were not kept private. Ancient cultures offered them to the dream community: for counsel, prophecy, or myth-making. In contrast, in our era, dreams often vanish with the sound of alarms, phone alerts, or morning news streams. They recognize that we are flooded with distractions, which compromise our ability to attend to dream life, which can only exist through active reflection.

They acknowledge that states of depression, loneliness, and meaninglessness are rising worldwide. This has been attributed to a loss of soul and a loss of belonging: to self, others, and the living world. Our mythology of separation has become epidemic. Willow and Eva show us how the process of cultivating dreams—an experience that transcends culture and language—can counter and restore this separation, which manifests in our lost connection to Self, others, the world, and the cosmos.

As doom scrolling and passive stream feeding numbs our imagination, dreamwork invites silence, slowness, and the reflective imagination—a practice rich with attentiveness. To apprentice dreaming is to reacquaint ourselves with soul—in service to Earth and to all beings.

May this book allow you to step into the world of dreaming and open yourself to your dreams—whatever form they take. In the sacred space between dream and listener, images live, emotional truths stir, and the soul speaks. This book is not a guide to *interpretation*. Instead, it is an invitation to a *relationship*. To join not only the authors, but also your dreaming self, in one of the oldest, most human, deeply soulful practices we can experience.

Helen Marlo, PhD
Dean, School of Psychology, and professor at Notre Dame de Namur University
Clinical psychologist (PSY 15318) and analyst member,
C. G. Jung Institute of San Francisco
Coeditor and contributing author, *The Spiritual Psyche in Psychotherapy: Mysticism, Intersubjectivity, and Psychoanalysis*

References

Bion, W. (1962). *Learning from experience*. Heinemann.
Grotstein, J. (1981). Wilfred Bion: The man, the psychoanalyst, the mystic—a perspective on his life and work. *Contemporary Psychoanalysis*, *17*(4), 501–504.
Grotstein, J. (2000). *Who is the dreamer who dreams the dream?* Routledge.

Jung, C. G. (1960). *The collected works of C. G. Jung: Vol. 8. The structure and dynamics of the psyche*, (R. F. C. Hull, Trans.; 2nd ed.). Princeton University Press. (Original work published 1954.)

Jung, C. G. (1964). *Man and his symbols*. Aldus Books.

Jung, C. G. (1969). Synchronicity: An acausal connecting principle. In *The structure and dynamics of the psyche* (R. F. C. Hull, Trans.; 2nd ed., Vol. 8). Princeton University Press. (Original work published 1952.)

Jung, C. G. (1988). *Nietzsche's Zarathustra: Notes of the seminar given in 1934–1939*. Princeton University Press.

Krippner, S., & Friedman, L. (2010). *Mysterious minds: The neurobiology of psychics, mediums, and other extraordinary people*. Praeger/ABC-CLIO.

Krippner, S., Ullman, M., & Honorton, C. (1971). A precognitive dream study with a single subject. *Journal of the American Society for Psychical Research*, *65*(2), 192–203.

Main, R. (2007). *Revelations of chance: Synchronicity as spiritual experience*. State University of New York Press.

Marlo, H. (2022). Experiencing the spiritual psyche: Reflections on synchronicity-informed psychotherapy. *Jung Journal: Culture & Psyche*, *16*(4), 44–69. https://doi.org/10.1080/19342039.2022.2125770

Merkur, D. (2010). James Grotstein and the transcendent position. In *Explorations of the psychoanalytic mystics*. Rodopi.

Mossbridge, J. A., Tressoldi, P., Utts, J., Ives, J. A., Radin, D., & Jonas, W. B. (2014). Predicting the unpredictable: Critical analysis and practical implications of predictive anticipatory activity. *Frontiers in Human Neuroscience*, *25*(8), 146. https://doi.org/10.3389/fnhum.2014.00146

Myers, F. W. H. (1943). *Human personality and its survival of bodily death* (L. H. Myers, Ed.). HardPress. (Original work published 1903)

Ogden, T. H. (2004). On holding and containing, being and dreaming. *International Journal of Psychoanalysis*, *85*(6), 1349–1364. https://psycnet.apa.org/doi/10.1516/T41H-DGUX-9JY4-GQC7

Schredl, M. (2009). *Frequency of precognitive dreams: Association with dream recall and personality variables. Journal of the Society for Psychical Research*, *73*(895[2])[2], 83–91.

Thalbourne, M. A., & Houran, J. (2000). Transliminality, the mental experience inventory and tolerance of ambiguity. *Personality and Individual Differences*, *28*(5), 853–863. https://doi.org/10.1016/S0191-8869(99)00143-9

Valášek, M., Watt, C., Hutton, J., Neill, R., Nuttall, R., & Renwick, G. (2014). Testing the implicit processing hypothesis of precognitive dream experience. *Consciousness and Cognition*, *28*, 113–125. https://doi.org/10.1016/j.concog.2014.06.011

ACKNOWLEDGMENTS

To my husband, Daniel Trimbach, for partnership in dreaming nondual love and living faith.

To Eva Tuschman Leonard, for dream companionship and living grace.

To Max Regan, for living presence across distance, and for always believing in me.

To my many teachers: family—including Kathy and Mark Pearson; Maurine and Al Trimbach; Scott, David, and Adam Pearson, and Kim Cusato; Ann, Kevin, Quinn, and Ryan Rice; and all the ancestors—friends; felines; colleagues; mentors; supervisors; students; supervisees; consultees; patients and therapists, expressly Catherine Seidel, for sharing this dream life in such meaningful ways.

Expressly, to my spiritual friends—teachers and colleagues—for welcoming dreams: Khenpo Tsültrim Gyamtso Rinpoche, Ari and Rose Goldfield, of/and Marpa Foundation; Lama Palden Drolma, Eric Ramstad, Annik Brunet, Vipassana Esbjorn-Hargens, of/and Sukhasiddhi Foundation; Ken Wilber, Roger Walsh, Sean Esbjorn-Hargens, James Baye, Susanne Cook-Greuter, Beena Sharma, Nicole Kieler Feagley, Nicole Churchill, Richard Munn, Mark Forman, Jonathan Reams, Adam Leonard, Corey Devos, Bonnie Bostrom, Ray and Victoria Greenleaf, Bruce Alderman, Layman Pascal, Patrick Sweeney, Don Milani, Sally Kempton, Sofia Diaz, Genpo Roshi, and Diane Hamilton, of/and the Integral mandala; Michael Eigen, James Grotstein, Robin Bagai, Stephen Bloch, and Ofra Eshel, of/and the Eigen workshop mandala, including Keri Cohen, Loray Daws, Shifa Haq, Shalini Masih, Adam Shechter, Ebru Salman, Stewart Morton, Mitchel Becker, Alitta Kullman, Paul DeBlassie III, Jeff Eaton, and Jani Santamaría; Helen Marlo and Notre Dame de Namur University; Sister Dolores Maguire, Father Roger Gustafson, and St. Hilary Church; Breck Waldman, Christina Bethke Rodgers, Nona Smolko, Bill Bickley, Christine Powell, Cynthia Sauer, Cynthia Stan Mellow, and Wilmington Friends School; Estelle Freedman, Susan Okin, Feminist, Gender, and Sexuality

Studies Program, Jamie Green, Elisabeth Osgood Campbell, Nina Farana, Marisa Nordstrom, and Everyday People, Stanford University; Frank Ostaseski and Zen Hospice Project; Dale Asrael, Laurie Rugenstein, Jane Carpenter Cohen, John Davis, Transpersonal Counseling Psychology and Music Therapy Programs, Naropa University; Claire Riley and Music Care Program, Boulder Community Hospital; Richard Freeman, Joanne Gatti, Tami Simon, and Yoga Workshop; Dzogchen Ponlop Rinpoche, Howard Aposhyan, and Nalandabodhi Seattle; Danelle Reed, Jennifer Decoteau, and Kwawachee Counseling Center of the Puyallup Tribal Health Authority; Diane Kaplan, Alan Kubler, Elisa Ambrosia, Sophie Wasson, Medical Hill Neurobehavioral Psychiatric Ward, California College of the Arts Counseling Center, the (former) Women's Therapy Center (of Berkeley), UCSF AIDS Health Project (now UCSF Alliance Health Project), and the Wright Institute; Beth Roosa, Denise Lew, and Psychological Services Center, Alliant International University, San Francisco; Rene Dumetz, Margaret Boucher, Lani Chow, David Cushman, Stephanie Chen, Christopher Dryer, Penelope Asay, Andrew Harlem, Frank Echenhofer, Tonya Dowding, Brian Lieske, Jonalyn Blaha, and Clinical Psychology PsyD Program, California Institute of Integral Studies; Ghazal Karimpour, *Fort Da*, and Northern California Society for Psychoanalytic Psychology; Jeffrey Moulton Benevedes, LeeAnn Pickrell, *Jung Journal: Culture & Psyche,* and the C. G. Jung Institute of San Francisco; Integral Relational Therapeutic Arts.

Willow Pearson Trimbach

To my husband, Adam Leonard, my earth angel, for companioning me through this mysterious and beautiful dream that is our life together.

To my parents, Mark and Jana Tuschman, who have cultivated my soul life from the beginning and nurtured it to flourish.

To my steadfast brother, Avi Tuschman, for always believing in me.

To my dear soul friend, Willow Pearson Trimbach, for being a compassionate and wise doula of my inner life.

To my mentor and friend, Anne Germanacos, for her ongoing curiosity and support of my creative endeavors.

To my teacher, Francis Weller, for accompanying and guiding my soul through the terrain of The Underworld.

To Naomi Mindelzun, my creative godmother, for always encouraging and uplifting my artistic life.

In memory of Judith Komoroske who was my first teacher of mysticism, poetry, and the beauty that moves the spirit.

Eva Tuschman Leonard

To Helen Marlo for your inspiring and prescient foreword.

To Jill Salberg, Melanie Suchet, Kate Hawes, Deepika Batra, Aakriti Aggarwal, and LeeAnn Pickrell, for vision and stewardship, from proposal, to review, to publication.

Willow Pearson Trimbach and Eva Tuschman Leonard

CREDITS

"Guru Bodhichitta," Unruffled Productions © 2012. Used with permission of the songwriters, Willow Pearson Trimbach and Eric Ramstad: *The Watermoons*.

"Tara's Promise," Unruffled Productions © 2012. Used with permission of the songwriters, Willow Pearson Trimbach and Eric Ramstad: *The Watermoons*.

INTRODUCTION

Learning from Dreaming

This book is for dreamers. Which is to say, this book is for everyone.

The intention of this book is to awaken *to* (not only from) the living dreams of the day and night that visit us, that compose our very being and becoming, which we in turn may attune to, may listen to, and may learn from. Such a practice of awakening *to* our dreams is a direct path of liberation, and this direct path is available to all.

The aspiration of this book is to be in conversation with these living dreams in order to deepen our relationship to ourselves, to others, to the world—the cosmos in which we live—the very fabric of our dreams.

The greatest myth that most people harbor about dreams is that dreams are not real. As this book will present and demonstrate, dreams are very real, in the sense that they communicate emotional truths. When we listen deeply to our dreams, we can hear those emotional truths, the messages of the soul. Perhaps this is a hidden meaning of the everyday wish that a given dream becomes a "dream come true."

Listening for those emotional truths incubated in dreams, in all of their complexity, is one of the core practices of learning from the mystery of the soul. This is how we hold our dreams in this book project, over and above any particular theoretical orientation or idea or any singular interpretation or even association.[1] In this book, we make room for all readings of the dream, all realizations of the dreamscape, in order to learn from this mystery.

Learning from dreams is continuous. Their essential mystery is unending. The view applied in this book is that dreams have their own subjectivity, their own phenomenology, their own beingness: we simply apprentice that dream subjectivity from our multiple intuitive perspectives, in the sense that we approach dreams as living mentors possessing deep knowledge we seek to learn. As we attune to them, dreams speak from the timeless living presence of the eternal now.

DOI: 10.4324/9781003591863-1

Yet, psychological theory, spiritual practice, artistic practice, relationships, communities, and cultures all shape our intuitive listening. These lenses of dreaming variously provide the helpful distancing and dissolution of depersonalization and derealization—the sense of unreality that allows for creating space and disengagement and can lead to the realization of illusion, joined together with attachment and embodiment. We engage witnessing and "withnessing" at once (Eshel, 2019b). Our listening is both informed and influenced by the presence of untold background realms, including relational psychoanalysis; Integral Theory, practice, and mandala (Esbjörn-Hargens, 2023; Pearson, 2014; Pearson Trimbach, 2022, 2023)[2]; family systems and transgenerational trauma (Salberg & Grand, 2017a, 2017b, 2024); Bionian psychoanalysis (expressly through James Grotstein, 2000, Michael Eigen, 2018, and Ofra Eshel, 2019b); the Eigen mandala (the community of scholar practitioners and laypeople who study, practice, apply, and further the work of psychoanalyst Michael Eigen[3]); Jungian analysis (Aizenstat, 2006, 2011; Bosnak, 2007; Jung, 1963, 2009; Sullivan, 2010); and transpersonal psychology (Brown, 2020; Pearson Trimbach, 2024a, for work on transpersonal psychoanalysis). We are also informed by music and song; painting and ceramics; meditation; relationships with people (family, friends, teachers, supervisors, therapists, students, clients/patients), with animals, with nature; and by the unseen (principally Buddhist, Jewish, Quaker, Christian Gnostic, Catholic, Metís Cree, ecumenical, and Integral spiritualities).

Combining and condensing these pathways of dreaming, we could say that the perspective of the dream simulcasts the intimacy of appearances, the dissolution of emptiness, and the possibility of openness. In receiving dreams, we allow ourselves to become radically unfamiliar. A portal to the radically unfamiliar, dreams usher us into contact with the deeper layers of being. Including and partnering with those deeper layers of being, we expand. In that expansion, we are in a process of realizing the nondual truths of Self/no-self (Almaas, 2014).

Taken together, these backgrounds and these variously foregrounded realms of theory, practice, relationships, and communities contribute to the formation of the *dreambody* (Mindell, 1998, 2009, 2014; Pearson, 2021), or third body, born through and born of our collaboration. The dreambody is a subtle body dimensionality of relationship (Cox, 2022), composed of the innermost relational layers of psychic presence, that expands and includes the physical body.

This book is neither an academic survey of dream theory, nor is it a guide for how to interpret your dreams. Rather, what interests us in this book is cultivating the practice of deeply listening to our dreams and how the dreambody comes alive through our shared reverence and reverie. By using narrative examples from our own dream life, we reveal our own longings, inquiries, reveries, and discoveries as we apprentice the emotional truths of dreaming, individually and in collaboration.

The further aspiration of this book is to inspire you to be in conversation with your own living dreams of the day and night that visit you—that compose your very being—to help you listen for them and attune to them—in solitude, in friendship, in artistry—in multiple modes of receptivity and reflection. The dream dialogues that unfold between us have been enriching and transformative, and we hope that they will inspire both clinicians and general readers to approach the life of dreams as a relational, living, psychotherapeutic, and spiritual practice. The purpose of this book is to inspire you to be in conversation with dreams you imagine, dreams you create, dreams you invent, dreams you discover—to learn from the mystery of the soul from which they emerge.

Living Emotional Truth

In honoring the life of dreams, it is important to center the confluences and distinctions between emotional experience and emotional truth. *Emotional truth* is a phrase drawn from psychoanalyst Wilfred Bion; "emotional truth" is a translation, on the personal level, of Bion's psychoanalytic symbol "O," itself connoting the unknown and unknowable, which we can yet become and in becoming we can yet realize. From an integral perspective, emotional experience, the life of feeling, is a gateway to the realizations of emotional truth. Yet, paradoxically, direct emotional truth[4] requires a path beyond that gate. Emotional truth itself is layered; it comes in waves. Emotional experiences have to be sifted through in order to source the treasures of the dreaming sea. Emotional experience is the raw material of emotional truth, but emotional truth is only sourced by listening for the latent wisdom harbored within the dream, beyond manifest displays. There are levels of emotional truth to be discerned, which can only be realized—sometimes gradually, sometimes suddenly—by making "contact with the depths" (to quote the title of a book by Michael Eigen).

The path is one of continual realizations, shining forth from multiple levels of development, yet only available to the level of development where we are presently stationed, as a temporal state of consciousness or an enduring stage of consciousness. As we demonstrate through these thirteen chapters, in the process of recording, reflecting on, conversing with, and dialoguing about dreams, we discover how to listen to these depths of the soul, the depths that shore us up and the depths that take us further into the unknown sea. As we swim that sea together, we hope to transmit something about the intuitive method of listening for and contacting the emotional truth of dreams. We become available to these layers of emotional truth, both their links and their disjunctures, as we home in on the profound emotional intelligence (as distinct from unreflective emotional reactivity) encoded and encrypted in the dream. It is a dream *practice*. In the process, blessed with a capacity to feel,[5] to be alive, we are touched by, as we ourselves touch, grace.

What do we mean when we speak of *grace*?

We are reminded of the words of the philosopher-poet John O'Donohue, in his book *Beauty: The Invisible Embrace*. O'Donohue writes, "What you encounter, recognize or discover depends to a large degree on the quality of your approach … When we approach with reverence, great things decide to approach us" (2004, pp. 23–24). O'Donohue notes that in many ancient cultures people practiced "careful rituals of approach. An encounter of depth and spirit was preceded by careful preparation" (p. 23). By embodying gentleness and patience, by eliciting curiosity and trust, we become fully available to receive the mysteries of our souls as communicated through the language of dreams.

We experience grace as this felt sense of reverence for the sacred that dwells in all that is.

We apprentice Grace, meaning that we both access and learn from Grace, by developing and deepening our relationship to the soul's divine gifts, opening ourselves to receive the mysterious and wondrous offerings of our dreamlife. New meanings, new questions, new revelations, whether mercurial, subtle, or awe-inducing, can only emerge through our growing awareness and receptivity to psyche's enigmatic expressions, the ever-unfolding poetry and plays of our dreams …

Apprenticeship to Dreaming

We began this work by initiating an apprenticeship to dreaming.

Although we met in 2014 in a postgraduate clinical training program in relational psychotherapy at the Women's Therapy Center in Berkeley, California, our footsteps had already trod along similar trails. We both earned our undergraduate degrees at Stanford University, albeit fifteen years apart in different programs, and later immersed ourselves in Buddhist practice, expressive arts and their therapeutic modalities, and eventually both found our way to The Wright Institute, also in Berkeley, California, for graduate studies in clinical psychology.

A shared passion for the creative process, the power of the unconscious, and devotion to spirituality threaded through our interests in the psyche. Eva is a visual artist and a ceramicist. And Willow is a musician, singer, songwriter, and music therapist. We have always had the connection of artistry—the healing arts and the expressive arts—as well as our study and practice in psychotherapy and meditation.

As our friendship evolved, our conversations moved away from the proverbial question *How are you?* and toward the question *How is your dream life?* And so, eventually our monthly check-in calls became invitations for each of us to share selected dream material that we held and explored in a sacred space between us. Intuition guided us as we learned to create an organic container for vulnerable, numinous, and enigmatic stories to be told. We developed a relational ritual that allowed us to witness one another's dream images with the utmost care, sensitivity, and curiosity. This book reveals the creative emergence of this practice as we learned to tend to our dream lives together (see Aizenstat, 2006, 2011).[6]

We started by creating an hour, about once every month or so, over a few years, to each share a dream that we recalled and sometimes wrote down. In that hour, we would bring a dream or dream fragment to relate and to give it voice. In the telling of the dream, both the dreamer and the dream partner would deeply listen, noting associations, questions, observations, intuitions, and heartfelt sense. Then, we would exchange these links and connections and wonderments, back and forth, as we allowed the dream to open further into our awareness and felt experience, to learn from the dream and its revelations of emotional truth as an expression of the mystery of the soul.

This process deepened, in each of us, the presence of our dreams, not only during the night but also in everyday life. Nighttime dreams and waking dreams began to be recognized as a continuous dreamscape. We opened an ear and listened for our dreams with the express possibility of sharing them with a trusted other who was also opening an ear to her dreamlife. Dreamlife—no longer relegated to the shadows—became an honored guest, an invited companion, welcomed into the light of awareness throughout the day and night.

We slowly started identifying dreams that we would select for the book project. Rather than having our conversations by phone, we started having them on Zoom, and we started recording those conversations and then transcribing them so that we could hear back and listen to and reread what we had discussed. Through that process, rather than having each of us share a dream across an hour, we started extending the time that we would give to each dream so we would spend an hour on one person's dream, and then the next dream session we would spend an hour on the other person's dream, and continue back and forth, month to month.

These conversations are between trusted friends, not psychotherapy sessions between a therapist and her patient, even as psychotherapeutic wisdom is drawn upon. These conversations are not intended to emulate the psychotherapeutic form, even as there are inevitably some similarities. Though we are both psychotherapists and we make use of psychological theory and academic scholarship to support our engagement, our frame is simply a willingness to be sensitive to Psyche's direct teachings and to be vulnerable with one another and learn from our own dreams as much as from one another's dreams. Our effort in this text is to translate theory into everyday language—both the theory that we use to describe a nuance of direct experience and the theory that we further or originate to reflect how we understand that direct experience. In this way, scholarship supports direct experience and participates in unfolding experience; yet, the conceptual realm does not lead the way, even as it quietly fosters and instrumentally accompanies the process.

Eventually, we selected specific dreams to include in the writing of this book. We followed an intuitive path in choosing dreams to apprentice—bringing to light the dreams that called out from the depths of the soul. This included dreams and nightmares. And at this juncture, we decided to include not only our nighttime dreams but also our waking dreams, linking these dimensions of being and becoming as conjoined portals of dreaming—throughout the day and night. In this way, we also sourced and curated artistic dreams—emanating from the continuity of day and night—of music/singing (through Willow) and image/painting (through Eva).

It's been very instructive, this process of listening for dreams that we wish to share, identifying and writing those upon waking, sharing them with one another through the recorded Zoom format, transcribing them, rereading them, and then working with them, individually, by reflecting on the dream dialogue further.

In this way, we've each extended the amount of physical time that we might give a dream ordinarily. We've incubated these dreams across many months and even beyond a year or more. That incubation has allowed us to learn more deeply from the dreams and, in that way, allowed the mystery of the dream to unfold, allowed the layers of the dream to deepen, and allowed the perspective of the soul to hold the various voices, images, identifications, and figures in the dream.

In that process, we found that each of our dream lives was deepening and that we were creating more space in our lives for our dreams. Then, too, we created an intentional space between us for sharing our dreams. Just knowing that there was this receptive space in trusted friendship where we could share our dreams with one another catalyzed psychic space to extend to our dream lives.

Apprenticeship to Grace

Dreams were never intended solely for the dreamer. In ancient cultures, dreams were offered into the collective as stories intended to be explored, interpreted, and uplifted together. Dreams could be prophesy, amplification of cultural myths, sources of potential wisdom. Relational practice allowed us as humans to share in this sacred ritual of tending to and learning from our dreams. And this learning, a reciprocally intimate learning about the transpersonal dimensions of dreams through the deeply personal dimensions of dreams and vice versa, was no less than a path of liberation.

In contemporary times, we've sadly lost touch with this communal practice; our dream lives are often shunted into the shadows, the residue of images quickly dissipating as we instantly turn our attention to app notifications, newsfeeds, and our email inbox as soon as our alarm goes off.

In a world clamoring for our attention, why give our attention to our dreams?

Rates of depression and anxiety are rising, along with suicidality, indicating an epidemic of loneliness in our society and an acute crisis of meaning-making. We are more connected than ever through the internet and social media, but at a fundamental level we feel disconnected—from ourselves, from others, from the living, breathing sentient natural world. We've lost touch with our deep interconnectedness. So much of our existential angst and despair arises from this false sense of separateness. Dreams invite us back into an ecology of interconnectedness. By apprenticing our dreams, we re-merge with all life forms and approach every element with reverence. In the dream realm, nothing is "other." Perhaps unfamiliar, but no longer "other" when apprenticed.

At a time in our history when we are passively receiving hundreds of images per day streamed through our smartphones, tablets, and computer screens, we've somehow become anesthetized to the imagination. Our minds expect to be entertained. It's all too easy to thoughtlessly reach for our phones to scroll through the content that others post and repost, offering quick stimulation, but ultimately leading to a kind of somnolent disengagement or disassociation.

In contrast, engaging in the imaginal is about deep, attentive listening in the here-and-now. This contemplative practice requires a degree of attunement through silence, patience, slowness, sensitivity, witnessing, and receptivity. This can be challenging in a world full of diversion and noise.

Apprenticing our dreams matters in a world where we have lost touch with soul. The intimacy that arises from truly paying attention allows us to stay in relationship to the mysterious, wild, decaying, regenerating, ever-changing *Anima Mundi,* or the soul of the world. If we neglect our relationship to our inner world, so, too, does our relationship to the outer world suffer. Now, more than ever, we need to reawaken to the cries of the sentient breathing Earth if we are to care for her and all beings relying on her for survival. What's more, including and extending beyond this earthly realm, dreams are contiguous with the entire cosmos in its ongoing births and deaths.

Dreams contain and are themselves contained by multiple wisdom traditions, touched by and touching Grace. Dreams are, at once, a "royal road to the unconscious," as Freud famously invoked; a conduit of Great Spirit, as indigenous wisdom transmits; a portal to our true nature, as Buddhism points out; and an emanation of God's divinity, as Judaism and contemplative Christianity recognize. All of these wisdom traditions figure in our dreams, support our dream dialogues, and are welcomed in this book.

Through an emergent apprenticeship, to our dream life and to one another, we began to hear the themes of our selected dreams. Foremost among these themes was the presence of Grace, not only in the content of the dreams but also in the companioning of our dream life through our connection to each other. By Grace, the dreams speak to the mystery of the soul—through a scream, a cry, song, art, time, love, death, divinity, animal companionship, otherness, music, illness, and life. And as we listened ever more deeply, sourcing the emotional truths harbored within those dreams, we discovered pathways of the soul's liberation.

How to speak of Grace? Grace itself is a mystery, and one that calls. We variously write of *Grace* and of *grace*, as, from an integral vantage, at times we invite a second-person (Grace) relationship or connection, and at other times, we express a third-person (grace) experience of the occasion, phenomenon, or realization. We also recognize the first-person embodiment of Grace—when she or he appears, or they appear, in name and form as the luminous Self/no-self. These "big three" perspectives are essential "caesuras of dreaming" (see Pearson, 2021; see Pearson Trimbach, 2023 for "dreaming the caesura"). Together they disclose the "O" of Grace—Bion's "O" or zero, that unitive at-one-ment beyond perspective that is paradoxically unknown and yet possible to realize—what I am calling, after Sara Bareilles, the *kaleidoscope heart*.[7] Perhaps grace cannot be known or grasped and yet can be touched and experienced directly—recognized through the innermost kaleidoscope heart of divine presence, none other than ordinary mind experiencing everyday life. To dream is to realize grace. And to realize grace is to attune to a moment, and to a path, of illumination and liberation.

The Grace of Dreaming

Through the grace of dreaming, the soul shifts from being a stranger to being a mystery, where we take refuge in what psychologist Robin Bagai has called the *creative unknown* (personal communication, July 8, 2023). Bagai (see 2023, 2026 for his engagement with Eigen's work) has also offered that "Our dreams look backwards and forwards [at once]; they are sources of potential new births" (Bagai, 2020).

These are meaningful dimensions of the grace of dreaming—the co-emergence and interbeing of past, present, and future in dreams, and dreams as sources of potential new births. We further muse on the links and disjunctures between dreaming and that which cannot yet be dreamed. The act of engaging in dream dialogue with a receptive dream partner is a practice of listening for emotional truth, itself an act of grace. To explore these dimensions, here are our chapter summaries.

We begin with Chapter 1, "Scream: Learning from Being Heard," a waking dream born through the artistry of psychotherapy and the depth of being heard by another in one's innermost cry through screaming. Willow recounts her first experience of being heard by another in the depth of her soul's cry, through psychotherapeutic voicework at the tender age of nineteen. Through this description of being heard at the level of the soul, beyond narrative renderings of pain and suffering in constructed language, the power of psychotherapeutic voicework is exemplified as a catalytic waking dream that echoes the sounds of birth, of trauma, of death, and of freedom. Through the process of listening to sound–emptiness–sound, expressions of tender and wrathful compassion are presenced as Tara of Buddhism, Mary of Christianity, and Kali of Hinduism (in her form as the lesser known Hindu/Buddhist goddess Chinnamunda/Chinnamasta). As catalyst for, container for, and commentary on these reflections, Ofra Eshel's (2019a) work on the "vanished last scream" is centered. Willow's reconnection with this therapist, thirty-three years later, is held in the context of synchronicities (Marlo, 2022), uncanny communications (Eshel, 2016), and the ways in which memories, held as waking dreams, can be the sources of potential new births.

We continue with another waking dream, in Chapter 2, "Watch: Learning from Time," where the dreamer links her maternal grandmother's life and love, her bodhisattva vow, and her wedding day as co-emergent expressions of the interbeing of past, present, and future. The dreamer explores how this mode of relating to time as a series of nested dreams—a dream, within a dream, within a dream, is itself a birth. A silver watch with diamond chips from Willow's beloved maternal grandmother is the central transformative object and guiding dream image linking Willow's developmental experiences of love, through connection to her maternal grandmother, taking the bodhisattva vow, and getting married.

We then hear in Chapter 3, "Song: Learning from Singing—Guru Bodhichitta," where the dream translates itself into music. Sharing the dream song, *Guru Bodhichitta*, from Willow's original music catalogue as *The Watermoons*, we learn from the innermost teaching of primordial wisdom and compassion aware of its own nature. Through the ultimate teacher, Awakened Heart, as bodhichitta can be translated, the singer as dreamer begins to hear her own voice and so, too, her life-affirming link to the heart of the cosmos. The relationship between singing and dreaming, as the conjoined external and internal voices of the soul echoing inside and outside at once, is illustrated. Through the resonant emotional truth of the lyrics set to music, the practice and fruition of meditation is sung into being, as a guide to dreaming.

Furthering the original artistry of dreams, we encounter in Chapter 4, "Alchemy of Soul: Learning from Creativity and the Unconscious," Eva's journey into the essence of dreaming as a creative process and the practice of art-making as an extension of dream life. The dialogue emphasizes the importance of honoring the "nondual un/conscious," where creative practice becomes a spiritual path toward individuation. Eva discusses how the mysteries of a dream can be lived onward and amplified through the formation and exploration of new images. The chapter advocates for embracing the mystery of the creative process, allowing it to transform and inform both waking and dream life, ultimately leading to a more integrated and fulfilling existence.

Then, attending to the apparent multiplicity of being, we receive in Chapter 5, "Others: Learning from Multiple Selves." Herein Willow explores the mystery that we are to ourselves, through a nighttime dream pointing to multiple dimensions of self in both hidden and lucid conversation with one another. The nighttime dream figures an ego ideal, a persecutor, and a breakdown. At first, the voice of the soul is not heard. Then, through dream dialogue and further dream reflection, the transcendent and emergent self comes into being, by recognizing, centering, and listening to the voice of the soul harbored and encrypted by the dream. What was "other," now apprenticed, becomes merely unfamiliar and, through practice, ultimately relatable. The importance of beginner's mind is contemplated vis-à-vis clinical work. And in the process, a method of the grace of dreaming is introduced—namely, the caesura of the *dream navel* and the *dream umbilicus*, two ideas introduced by Sigmund Freud (2010) in his 1899 *Interpretation of Dreams*.

And in Chapter 6, "Surrender: Learning from Illness," we hear messages from the soul through the pain and struggle of long-term unresolved illness. Eva explores how approaching life as a kind of waking nightmare is the soul's medicine path when apprenticed. She conjures the Buddhist concept of emptiness and the notion that "life is but a dream" as a helpful orientation for co-existing with physical pain and that which is confusing and unknown. Eva examines how Psyche offers an infinite portal for liberation through our nighttime dreams no matter how constrictive the limitations of one's waking life, due to disability, illness, war, or imprisonment.

In Chapter 7, "Wanting Out: Learning from Cats—Bardo and the Shoji Screen," we hear further reflections on the life of the soul through listening to the adventures of cats. Bardo, Willow's indoor cat, desperately wants to get outside. This short waking dream illustrates the desire in us all to go beyond the boundaries of this life and the dance of taking this yearning to its edge, as we recognize how the soul is simultaneously bounded, through embodiment, and transcendent, through the spiritual psyche. The emergence of Bardo's path of kidney disease, and caring for her through the last stages of life, centers lived revelations of our conjoined immanence and transcendence.

In Chapter 8, "Circle Game: Learning from Cats—Chief and His Exercise Wheel," we witness the circle of life through a cat running on his exercise wheel. This simple beholding of a cat expressing his playful aliveness and, later in life, his "going on being," becomes one of turning toward Grace in all her mystery. At first, watching him is like a dizzy spell. Then he hits his stride in a steady hum, flying in the sky, even as the ground disappears beneath his paws, his feline body indigenous to the motion of stillness. This expanded description is the essence of Willow's orange tabby Abyssinian cat, Chief, running his "circle game" (to invoke a famous Joni Mitchel song)—his favorite activity—on the large black exercise wheel with a leopard patterned interior. Through this feline play, a metaphoric rotation on the wheel of life is expressed simultaneously and variously as repetitive and routine, as tentative and quizzical, and as opening to the never-before-never-again novelty of the present moment waking dream, from opening to life as it is. Holding these various views, within the circle of being, is one of many gifts of learning from cats.

With Chapter 9, "Devotion: Learning from Nondual Love," the advent of union between souls is centered, with reflections on four of Willow's precious teachers: Khenpo Tsültrim Gyamtso Rinpoche, Lama Palden Drolma, Ken Wilber, and Michael Eigen. Through a dream of her Buddhist Rinpoche, through a dream of her Lama, through a dream of philosopher Ken Wilber—her integral mentor—and the Integral mandala, and through a dream of her psychoanalytic mentor, Michael Eigen, Willow goes into the very heart of these ever-evolving relationships, demonstrating how we live in one another, through the life of the soul, communicated in dreams. The interbeing of dreaming is centered through the individual and interpersonal lenses of these kindred nighttime dreams between student and teacher. Through this dreaming nondual love (Almaas, 2023a, 2023b), Eshel's (2016, 2019c), "delving into the profound mystery of telepathy at the heart of clinical psychoanalysis" as uncanny communication is extended to student/teacher/mandala experience.

Through Chapter 10, "Departure: Learning from Goodbye," we hear the midwifery of being through dying. Eva shares with us her journey in accompanying her soon-to-be father-in-law at the threshold of death, on a long-distance phone call as her father-in-law takes his last earthly breath from his hospice bed. Eva reflects on the radical presencing in the here-and-now that is required for entering the liminal state between life and what lies beyond the veil. Being with the ultimate mystery and the great unknown unfolds as a collective dream experience for all who are present.

Then, with Chapter 11, "Burial: Learning from Death—Île-à-la-Crosse," we cross the threshold of being on the other side of life. Here we learn from a nighttime dream, about a transcultural practice of caring for the dead by invoking burial rituals of two tribes that are in conflict. Willow explores a nighttime dream about "new Île-à-la-Crosse." In "real life," Île-à-la-Crosse is a place in present-day Saskatchewan, Canada. It is the geographic location of the marriage of Willow's great-great-great-great-grandfather and grandmother.[8] The contemporary landscape of war, foremost among them war between Russia and Ukraine, and the war between Israel and Hamas, contextualizes this dreaming the collective cry of the world soul—a cry for understanding across and among cultural groups. Transgenerational trauma centers the conversation (Salberg & Grand, 2017a, 2017b, 2024). Listening for caesura's cry serves as catalyst for, container for, and commentary on dreaming a "new Île-à-la-Crosse" (Eshel, 2022). "War as a means of cross-fertilization" is invoked (personal communication, Michael Eigen online seminar, April 30, 2024). Apprenticing Grace, in apprenticing the dream, appears in the form of Dream Blessing through Catholic and indigenous (Metís Cree and Zuni) lineages.

In Chapter 12, "Ascension: Learning from Divinity," we consider embodiment as an instrument of spirit and contemplate its release back to the groundless ground of being. Willow relates a nighttime dream of Christ's ascension, in which Hercules (a strong man) and Jane (a feminist artist) figure centrally, inviting equal regard for each figure and how they illuminate and also foil one another. The *chuppah*, a traditional Jewish wedding tent, offering hospitality and protection, to welcome God's blessing through the union of souls, created the space for this dream incubation and emergence. The chuppah figures here as a refuge, gestating an invocation of this nighttime dream. The nested dreams presented here are written as a prequel, a nighttime dream, a postscript, and an afterword …

Lastly, in Chapter 13, "Grace: Learning from Living—Tara's Promise," we listen for the co-emergent presence of here, there, somewhere, nowhere, and everywhere, through the expression of music as dreaming,[9] as "Tara's Promise," a song from Willow's original music catalogue as *The Watermoons* dedicated to the Noble Lady Tara.[10] The relationship between the Buddhist deity Tara and the universal revelations of grace as moments of opening to the soul and as paths of liberation, supported by Jung's synchronicity (Marlo, 2022), are uncovered. Willow's nighttime dream of Eva, an expression of the spiritual psyche (Pearson & Marlo, 2021), figures *dreaming soul* and *touching grace.* Dreaming this demonstrates and transmits Tara's "appearance–emptiness–appearance," "sound–emptiness–sound," and the "clarity–emptiness–thought" of co-dreaming (Haq & Masih, 2018), through nested dreams, dreaming's reach, and the simulcast of dreams. In this way, honoring the mystery of the soul, the grace of dreaming is realized as none other than the dreaming of Grace.

Dreaming Grace

In the process of writing this book, through an apprenticeship to the grace of dreaming, we began to recognize that, in a meaningful sense, we are also dreaming grace. In other words, the grace of dreaming is a reciprocal process. Like the famous

Esher image of the hand drawing itself, dreaming is a process of emergent being that renders the absolute subjectivity of being itself. We hope that the chapters that follow offer a felt, direct, experiential sense of how, at root, the grace of dreaming is, at once, the dreaming of grace. The discovery of grace seeds Grace's ongoing emergence and emanation.

We hope that through the illustration and transmission of our own apprenticeship to our dreams, you might also be inspired to take up this call, in your own creative ways, to honor your own soul and its presence in and contributions to the world, and to the cosmos—the planets and the stars, space itself, and all who experience the rhythms of birth and death. On the path of inquiry, we behold and explore the links and disjunctures between dreaming and that which cannot yet be dreamed. Perhaps we might discover together, in our exchange, that we are dreaming Grace into being through our discernment of emotional truth …

Notes

1 "Learning from…, the framework for this book, its title, and each chapter's title, is in the lineage of psychoanalyst Wilfred Bion, who wrote *Learning from Experience* (1962) (2024).
2 See Pearson Trimbach (2022, 2023) for creative emergence between relational psychoanalysis and integral psychology as Integral Relational theory and practice; see Pearson (2014) for work on *Dreaming Integral*.
3 See Bloch and Daws (2015); Cohen and Daws (2024); Daws (2023); Daws and Cohen (2024); Eaton (2011); Fuchsman and Cohen (2021); Pearson Trimbach (2024b).
4 See Grotstein (2000) for a formulation of a "truth drive," which evolved from Bion's work.
5 See Eigen (2024) on the "Pain of No Pain."
6 See S. Aizenstat's work on dream tending for a luminous view of and relationship to dreaming. Willow has worked with Aizenstat's book *Dream Tending* (2006, 2011), together with his audio program by the same name, for several years; she teaches Aizenstat's work, together with her own work, in her transpersonal course at the California Institute of Integral Studies.
7 See S. Bareilles, *Kaleidoscope Heart* [album], produced by Neal Avron for Epic Records, 2010.
8 For context on Charlotte Small Thompson, a Metís Cree woman, and her marriage to David Thompson, an Englishman who immigrated to Canada, see Pearson Trimbach (2022).
9 See S. Bloch (2024).
10 Hear the song "Tara's Promise" by the Watermoons (Willow Pearson and Eric Ramstad) at www.lionessroars.org/music/redboat as well as through Apple Music, SoundCloud, Spotify, and other downloadable and streaming music services worldwide.

References

Aizenstat, S. (2006). *Dream tending: Techniques for uncovering the hidden intelligence of your dreams* [Audiobook]. Sounds True.
Aizenstat, S. (2011). *Dream tending: Awakening to the healing power of dreams*. Spring Journal Books, Inc.
Almaas, A. H. (2014). *Runaway realization: Living a life of ceaseless discovery*. Shambhala.

Almaas, A. H. (2023a). *Love unveiled: Discovering the essence of the awakened heart.* Shambhala.
Almaas, A. H. (2023b). *Nondual love: Awakening to the loving nature of reality*. Shambhala.
Bagai, R. (2020). Emotional Storm Seminar [Video course on the work of Michael Eigen], November 11. Used with permission from *RobinBagai.com*.
Bagai, R. (2023). *Commentaries on the work of Michael Eigen: Oblivion and wisdom, madness and music*. Routledge.
Bagai, R., Ed. (2026). *A Michael Eigen companion: Moments of wisdom from a psychoanalytic mystic*. Routledge.
Bion, W. (2024). *Learning from experience*. Routledge.
Bloch, S. (2024). Music as dreaming. In K. Cohen & L. Daws (Eds.), *Primary process impacts and dreaming the undreamable object in the work of Michael Eigen: Becoming the welcoming object*. Routledge.
Bloch, S., & Daws, L. (Eds.). (2015). *Living moments: On the work of Michael Eigen*. Routledge.
Bosnak, R. (2007). *Embodiment: Creative imagination in medicine, art and travel*. Routledge.
Brown, R. S. (2020). *Groundwork for a transpersonal psychoanalysis: Spirituality, relationship, and participation*. Routledge.
Cohen, K. S., & Daws, L. (Eds.). (2024). *Toxic nourishment and damaged bonds in the work of Michael Eigen: Working with the obstructive object*. Routledge.
Cox, S. (2022). *The subtle body: A genealogy*. Oxford University Press.
Daws, L. (2023). *Michael Eigen: A contemporary introduction*. Routledge.
Daws, L., & Cohen, K. (Eds.). (2024). *Primary process impacts: Dreaming the undreamable object in the work of Michael Eigen. Becoming the welcoming object*. Routledge.
Eaton, J. (2011). *A fruitful harvest: Essays after Bion*. The Alliance Press.
Eigen, M. (2018). *The challenge of being human*. Routledge.
Eigen, M. (2024). The pain of no pain. *Psychoanalysis and Culture*, *46*(77). https://doi.org/10.5935/0101-3106.v46n77.11
Esbjörn-Hargens, S. (2023). *Types of nonduality and framework for varieties of nonduality* [handout]. Metaintegral Academy.
Eshel, O. (2016). In search of the absent analyst: Commentary on Janine de Payer's "uncanny communication. *Psychoanalytic Dialogues*, *26*(2), 185–197.
Eshel, O. (2019a). The vanished last scream: Winnicott and Bion. *Psychoanalytic Quarterly*, *88*(1), 111–140. https://doi.org/10.1080/00332828.2019.1558876
Eshel, O. (2019b). *The emergence of analytic oneness: Into the heart of psychoanalysis*. Routledge.
Eshel, O. (2019c). Would clinical psychoanalysis shy away from delving further into the unknown? On the mystery of telepathic dreams. *International Journal of Psychoanalysis*, *100*(3), 608–610. https://doi.org/10.1080/00207578.2019.1590121
Eshel, O. (2022). Bion's long road towards intuiting the patient's suffering: "Theoretical" vs. "Clinical. *Contemporary Psychoanalysis*, *58*(1), 46–76. https://doi.org/10.1080/00107530.2022.2083424
Freud, S. (2010). *The interpretation of dreams: The complete and definitive text* (J. Strachey, Trans.). Basic Books.
Fuchsman, K. & Cohen, K. S. (2021). *Healing, Rebirth and the Work of Michael Eigen: Collected Essays on a Pioneer in Psychoanalysis*. Routledge.
Grotstein, J. (2000). *Who is the dreamer who dreams the dream? A study of psychic presences*. The Analytic Press.
Haq, S., & Masih, S. (2018). Waiting in the dark. In M. H. Williams & M. Botbol Acreche (Eds.), *Counterdreamers: Analysts reading themselves* (pp. 81–90). The Harris Meltzer Trust, Karnac Books.
Jung, C. G. (1963). *Memories, dreams, reflections*. Pantheon Books.

Jung, C. G. (2009). *The red book: Liber novus.* (S. Shamdasani, Ed.) (S. Shamdasani, M. Kyburz, & J. Peck, Trans.). W. W. Norton & Co.
Marlo, H. (2022) Experiencing the spiritual psyche: Reflections on synchronicity-informed psychotherapy. *Jung Journal: Culture & Psyche*, *16*(4), 44–69, https://doi.org/10.1080/19342039.2022.2125770
Mindell, A. (1998). *Dreambody: The body's role in revealing the self.* Lao Tse Press.
Mindell, A. (2009). *Coma: The dreambody near death.* Lao Tse Press.
Mindell, A. (2014). *Working with the dreaming body*. CreateSpace Independent Publishing Platform.
O'Donohue, J. (2004). *Beauty: The invisible embrace*. Harper Perennial.
Pearson, W. (2014). Dreaming integral. *Journal of Integral Theory and Practice*, *9*(2), 162–168.
Pearson, W. (2021). Caesuras of dreaming: Being and becoming, thinking and imagining. In W. Pearson & H. Marlo (Eds.), *The spiritual psyche: Mysticism, intersubjectivity, and psychoanalysis* (pp. 180–201). Routledge.
Pearson, W. & H. Marlo (2021). *The spiritual psyche in psychotherapy: Mysticism, intersubjectivity, and psychoanalysis.* Routledge.
Pearson Trimbach, W. (2022). Integral relational practice of dreaming the caesura. Part 1: Opening further through the spiritual psyche. Part 2: Dreaming Charlotte Small Thompson. *Jung Journal: Culture & Psyche*, *16*(4), 115–123.
Pearson Trimbach, W. (2023). Psyche's score: The music of the integral psychodynamic sphere and its orbits. *Integral Review*, *18*(1), 254–277. https://integral-review.org/issues/vol_18_no_1_pearson_trimbach_psyches_score_music_of_the_integral_psychodynamic_sphere_and_its_orbits.pdf
Pearson Trimbach, W. (2024a). On the way to the altar: An illustration of transpersonal psychoanalytic psychotherapy. *International Journal of Transpersonal Studies*, *43*(1). https://digitalcommons.ciis.edu/advance-archive/84
Pearson Trimbach, W. (2024b). Welcoming dreams. In L. Daws & K. Cohen (Eds.), *Primary process impacts and dreaming the undreamable object in the work of Michael Eigen: Becoming the welcoming object*. Routledge.
Salberg, J., & Grand, S. (Eds). (2017a). *Trans-generational trauma and the other: Dialogues across history and difference*. Routledge.
Salberg, J., & Grand, S. (Eds). (2017b). *Wounds of history: Repair and resilience in the trans-generational transmission of trauma*. Routledge.
Salberg, J., & Grand, S. (2024). *Transgenerational trauma: A contemporary introduction.* Routledge.
Sullivan, B. S. (2010). *The mystery of analytical work: Weavings from Jung and Bion.* Routledge.

1

SCREAM

Learning from Being Heard

In this first chapter of the book, we begin with a waking dream born through the artistry of psychotherapy. Willow recounts her first experience of being heard by another in the depth of her soul's cry, through psychotherapeutic voicework at the tender age of nineteen. Through this description of being heard at the level of the soul, beyond narrative renderings of pain and suffering in constructed language, the power of psychotherapeutic voicework is experienced as a catalytic waking dream that echoes the sounds of birth, of trauma, of death, and of freedom. Her reconnection with this same therapist, thirty-three years later, opens her to the unceasing screaming of the world. This is juxtaposed with Eva's nighttime dream of learning to trust her own mind.

Prequel: In the Presence of the Dream

Eva: Yesterday I was reviewing your dream about meeting with your Tibetan Buddhist teacher (in Chapter 9, "Devotion: Learning from Nondual Love"). Vehicles appeared in the beginning and then in the middle of your dream.

Following that review, I had a dream that I just awoke from a few hours ago. It took place at night.

I went to a Buddhist meditation center with [my husband] Adam. I believe he said it was Shambhala.[1] The teacher who was facilitating was quite strict and had us standing in regimented rows. At a certain point this teacher came over to adjust me into a more upright position and I found it very off-putting. I departed in haste from Shambhala and got into a vehicle. But oddly, I was driving the vehicle from the passenger side seat using only my mind. There was no steering wheel and no one

DOI: 10.4324/9781003591863-2

in the driver's seat. In the dark, I got out of the car and found another vehicle—this time, a bicycle. I was bicycling through the night and trying to find my way back home.

Willow: What was it like riding the bicycle?

Eva: For me, it was a bit exhilarating because I haven't been able to ride a bicycle in many years. It felt really freeing and exciting and also a little scary because it was nighttime.

Willow: And what was it like to drive the car with your mind from the passenger seat?

Eva: Initially, I was concerned about how the car would have any control if no one was in the driver's seat. But soon I realized that I could trust my mind to navigate—even as it felt uncomfortable and definitely strange to wonder, "Should someone be in the driver's seat? Where is the wheel?" And then I thought, "Oh, well, that's appropriate because in many of the teachings of Buddhism, it's your consciousness that is the only thing you can control or change."

Willow: Or direct.

Eva: Or direct. Yes.

Willow: Or partner.

Eva: Yes, "partner" is better than "control." I fled a meditation session where I felt controlled by the master teacher, so I chose to get into my own vehicle.

Willow: Lovely. Thank you for sharing this present dream. Let's transition to the "scream" dream and listen in for how these two dreams may be connected since they are appearing in this nested way, with your present dream arising in response to my "Devotion: Learning from Nondual Love" dream series in Chapter 9 and in prequel to our dialogue centered on this waking dream of "Scream: Learning from Being Heard."

Eva: Thanks for listening, Willow, to this dream "hot off the press."

Willow: It's so apropos.

Thank you for speaking this present dream. It feels supremely relevant and is the first movement of our dialogue today.

Evolution from a Scream to a Dream[2] and The Vital Root of Compassion

Here is a waking dream, arising now in memory from thirty-five years ago …

At nineteen, I entered into therapy with Catherine Seidel, who was then a graduate student at the California Institute of Integral Studies (CIIS). I was an undergraduate student at Stanford. A dear friend, Nina Farana (see Chapter 11, "Burial:

Learning from Death—Île-à-la-Crosse") had recommended Catherine to me. Nina had intuited a potential therapeutic connection, as Catherine was both a singer and a horse whisperer, and Nina knew firsthand of my deep love of song and cats. Indeed, a mutual recognition of and participation in our indivisible transcendent and primal nature shaped the emergent therapeutic connection between Catherine and me.

Catherine would drive from San Francisco to Palo Alto, so we could meet on the Stanford campus. I would reserve one of the soundproof practice rooms in the music department for our sessions. As a therapist in training and as a vocal artist, Catherine and I met in the realm of what the Buddhists, according to a three-vehicle Vajrayana view,[3] called *sound–emptiness–sound*[4]—which can be translated as sound recognized as music, on the other side of and imbued with infinite silence. With Catherine's warm, steady, compassionate, and reliable presence—a conduit for boundless compassion and luminous presence, the likes of which the Buddhist deity Tara and the Christian presence of Mary possess—I screamed,[5] for an hour at a time across many weeks. I groaned and growled, wailed and cried. It was as if I were uttering lifetimes of pain. The rhythm of our sessions would move from tentative trust to exploratory utterances, gradually expanding to guttural groans that shook my foundation loose. Catherine was a steadfast support, both silently and through gentle, nonintrusive minimal encouragement, allowing me to scream from the depths. She heard me, as I felt my way through the rage and sorrow that had no beginning and no end. And yet, as *samsara*—the pain of beginningless time—moved through me, in rage against birth and death, there was a freedom in its passage, transcending mind. Being together was heartening. Catherine's intuitive capacity to receive and release, receive and release, receive, resonate, and release, in the basic space of awakened heart, touched my soul and sheltered it with unspeakable tenderness—the way that Tara and Mary do in the presence of Kali,[6] the goddess of creative destruction now unleashed.

What began as unutterable and unbearable pain became, in Catherine's presence, relatable, felt communication. For the first time, the pain of samsara now had a recognized voice. Kali music flowed.

I was heard on the level of my soul.

The impact of Catherine's natural presence, as a conduit of boundless compassion, re-appeared in my search for a therapist thirty-five years later. I wondered who I could turn to for support?

Catherine, who I had not been in contact with since I was in my twenties, popped into my mind. Was she still in practice, I wondered? I did a search on LinkedIn. And I was heartened to discover that she remained in practice, in Portola Valley (a city I had lived in for a year when I was seven years old). I took a chance and reached out. Yes, she could see me by Zoom! I was overjoyed to reconnect many lifetimes later.[7]

The work now takes a different shape between us. There have been further and more intense silent screams along the way, Kali ever-present, and yet that foundation of *sound–emptiness–sound* remains. Echoes of *sound–emptiness–sound* are teaching me still. This is the ever-ongoing learning of being heard in the scream—sounded or silent, like a bell that resounds in the radiant openness of Tara's, of Mary's, and of Kali's awakened heart, indivisible. This was the beginning of a timeless evolution from screaming to dreaming and the beginning reckoning with their basic rhythm.

Recalling this time in my life is, as my teacher Khenpo Tsültrim Gyamtso Rinpoche says, "like a dream when you know you are dreaming." It shines in my heart as a precious jewel of true connection that transcends time or place. It continues to resound in my being and becoming, itself like a waking dream when I know I am dreaming, resting still.

Hearing and Feeling This Rhythm of Screaming to Dreaming

There is a teaching in psychoanalysis that is a root work in every therapy, every analysis: to listen for and to hear the muted scream (Eshel, 2019) and interrupted cry (Ogden, 2006) of each patient as a groundwork of and for healing. This requires the clinician to begin to hear their own muted scream, their own interrupted cry, in order to unlock the flow of their emotional life. This allows them to resonate with a patient's emotional truths and—extending beyond any one individual, self, or other—to hear the scream, the cry, of the world. Eaton (2015) says that there is a scream that keeps on screaming and that as we tune into this frequency of emotional life on a collective level, we also may begin to then hear the rhythm of faith that, in the fashion of Bion, partners catastrophe as a convergence with faith. In my work with Catherine at age nineteen, I accessed my personal scream; in continuing with her now at age fifty-four, I am present to the screaming of the world, which puts me in touch with the scream that is heard, allowing me to partner the scream that keeps on screaming—albeit in new keys of silence and music and language. All of this is in concert with a faith that keeps on opening, transmuting, and transforming that screaming-to-dreaming. Writing this book is an embrace of the co-emergence of catastrophe and faith,[8] where screaming and dreaming realize one another as the throat and the ear of the Awakened Heart, a union of Tara, Mary, and Kali.

Afterward: In the Presence of the Dream

Willow: Let me just say that while Kali is the more familiar goddess of destruction-into-creation, I have known her as Chinnamunda/Chinnamasta,[9] which is a Hindu and, later, a Buddhist dream body of the deity. (The *dream-body* is a subtle dimensionality of psychic presence that expands and includes the physical body.) Chinnamunda/Chinnamasta is kindred to Kali, a particular form of Kali. She is somebody who visited me in my dream life in my late thirties, and I have followed the thread of her presence in psyche ever since. Chinnamunda/Chinnamasta is part of this dance of transcendence/immanence that we tap into with different deities, from different faith traditions, some well-known and others more hidden.

Chinnamunda/Chinnamasta transcends ego and inhabits it. Through her embodiment of destruction-into-creation, she is a conduit for embracing wrathful compassion. Once a stranger, according to Chinnamasta/Chinnamunda's realization, wrathful compassion becomes an ally and friend. By her hand, the ego surrenders to and now serves the Self/no-self.

Chinnamunda/Chinnamasta wears a garland of skulls like Kali, symbolizing the confrontation with one's own death and then integrating an acceptance of death and disappearance as indivisible dimensions of the cycles of life, rebirth, and renewal. She has a chopper in one hand—a large, curved blade, symbolizing cutting through delusion. She holds her own head, by her hair, in another hand. This symbolizes many realities, including her capacity for listening to intuition, listening from the un/conscious, listening beyond ego, and including yet transcending intellectual thought. From the opening of her neck flows three streams of blood. The middle stream goes to the mouth of her severed head. She then nourishes her ego with her own lifestream, now an ornament of emptiness. Ego now serves as a vehicle for ever-awakening being and becoming, expressing an integral desire for personal, interpersonal, and transpersonal emotional truth. And the other two streams of blood go to two other goddesses that are at her feet, themselves dancing on lotuses, symbolizing awakening. These are the embodiments of tantric couples, symbolizing the indivisibility of *samsara* (suffering) and *nirvana* (liberation).

She too is dancing on the lotus flowering of a tantric couple. She has snakes around her waist, which symbolize reckoning with the emotional truth of aversive emotions (Pearson, 2021), and a translucent tiger skin, symbolizing fearlessness. She dances within a ring of fire, demonstrating the illusory nature of this world and the mind that it is created in, with, and through, even as it vividly appears.

Embracing her has unleashed a deeper, silent, echoing, cosmic scream in me—the silent calamitous sounding of samsara (suffering) throughout the reaches of space, the likes of which I couldn't have fathomed a capacity to be present to at age nineteen, even as it visited me.

I think as I first wrote this chapter, with the book in mind, there was a desire to come to completion as if that screaming that arose at nineteen was held, heard, resolved, integrated, and so wouldn't happen again. As if personal healing was an end goal.

I think that was an illusion woven into the beginning of writing this chapter and maybe in some sense this book. The deeper order of teaching of the presencing of Tara, also as Mary, and Chinnamunda/Chinnamasta, also as Kali, is that the capacity for facing the scream and conducting the scream of samsara is something that continues without end. Both Mary and Chinnamunda/Chinnamasta demonstrate a recognition that the scream of samsara-and-nirvana-inseparable is a single scream, echoed in different keys, one expressed through the music of a gentle, tender love and one voiced through the music of a very fierce, wrathful love.

Eva: That fierceness and that rage, like a fountain, can emerge from a place of deep justice or a sense of deep injustice, which emerges from a place of deep love. We scream to protect what we care for most in this lifetime. We don't have enough representation in our contemporary Western culture of what that looks like—that fierce, feminine, rageful, feral, wild kind of love. Because it's so gory, visceral, and even grotesque, and yet it is so powerful that the blood is dripping on the tantric lovers on their lotus. It's an incredible transmission.

Willow: Her dismemberment is the seed and root of her union. She takes her own head, and this is no simplistic martyrdom. No act of masochism. This is no self-abnegation. This is a radical opening to all of life and death that embraces dissolution and transfiguration. This is the clear recognition that her lifestream feeds wherever she directs her attention—or has the potential to—and that lifeforce is at one with her lifeforce.

Eva: I'm glad you're saying that this isn't a simplistic martyrdom, or masochism, guarding against that misunderstanding of her. This feels like a vivid expression of *nondual love* (love that dissolves any separation between subject and object). I am really struck that, as such a young psychotherapist in training, Catherine trusted herself or trusted the process enough to give you space to express the multiplicity of that emotional truth.

Willow: As living images in the waking dream, I love the paradox that the room we screamed in was *soundproof* and, at the same time, that it was in the *music department*.

Eva: Right. Silence contained and held the scream.

Willow: There's something even in that scream that's unutterable. There's no bottom to the well of that scream. There's no end to it, and yet there absolutely was, and is, the experience of being heard that is life-changing.

Eva: I wrote that down: "She heard me. I was heard on the level of my soul." And what else could we ask for in a psychotherapeutic experience? "I was heard on the level of my soul." To me, that's the ultimate wish, the ultimate consummation of purposeful, meaningful psychotherapy: to feel heard on the level of the soul. Soul needed to speak, not through language and narrative, but through screaming, through guttural moaning.

And how incredible would it be if every young woman had that opportunity, had that space, had that witness?

Willow: It strikes me that as a person who doesn't have biological children of her own, that this experience with Catherine was a kind of birth process.

Eva: Yes. Absolutely.

Willow: It was like she attended my labor.

Eva: Yes.

Willow: And she was very much a midwife to my soul in that sense. And is.

Eva: A friend of mine was just laboring for five days and had an amazing doula by her side. And what she described of the birthing days feels very resonant with what you've just conveyed: that primal, guttural moaning that is necessary for new life to emerge, whether it's a literal child emerging out of the womb or the birthing of one's soul into a new iteration of self. I think it was Eric Fromm (1994) who said that "man's main task in life is to give birth to himself ..." How meaningful to think of Catherine as your attendant or doula or midwife.

I'm also reflecting on the fact that I too was a freshman at Stanford at one point in time, and I ended up leaving in the middle of my freshman year. I went abroad on my own, which was an extremely transformative period in my life of finally doing something that was self-authored and not based on other people's expectations of me. But I think if I had had a midwife like Catherine to witness my own version of the scream, I may not have had to leave school. But I was so used to being the "good student," the "good daughter," the "good girl" that I didn't have a place where I could unleash my own pain, anger, sadness, and aggression. How different it might have been had someone been there to witness and contain that. Even now, in my forties, I would like that experience. But at eighteen I experienced a very deep depression instead. The depression was a symptom of not being able to express and channel a scream that needed to be heard.

I don't think I was conscious that a scream needed to be unleashed; instead, I shut down and couldn't follow through with my schoolwork and needed to take a leave of absence. The psychologist who I sought help from at the student center was quick to prescribe medications. I knew that this was a soul's cry that didn't need anesthetizing. But there was no one to hear the cry and so I chose to leave. And I wonder, what would it be like if there were these soundproof rooms and these doulas available to hear the soul's cry?

Certainly there's a place for medication, but I think in my situation, I really needed a witness in the way Catherine was a witness for you. Most young people who come to Stanford and similar institutions are highly composed; what Catherine was offering you was a place to be decomposed, to dissolve, to be disillusioned and despairing. I love that you had the space to completely disintegrate, to become deranged. Especially as young women are expected to be hyperarranged.

Willow: That is music to my ears to hear that echo. Not a place to be composed, but a place to disintegrate. Not a space to be arranged, but a space to be allowed to be deranged. She invited the wildness in me to be brought to the airwaves in a way that was welcomed. She welcomed my madness as basic sanity. She had a faith that such welcoming would do its own soul work. I was able to partner this faith in the process.

Eva: Absolutely. I imagine that it was a seminal therapy in your young adult life and maybe the seeds were sewn that eventually led you on your path to now be a professor and clinical training director at CIIS, the school where Catherine was then in training. That's a pretty remarkable trajectory and a full-cycle movement.

Willow: And I think it says something about mandalas at work. In this book, in many ways we are exploring the experience of teaching mandalas. As we talked about in discussing the book's afterword, I was curious to learn that another definition of mandala is "a dream image." There are many definitions of mandala, and there are healing mandalas and teaching mandalas that can be one and the same collective dreambody. Certainly CIIS, where I currently teach and where Catherine was a student of psychotherapy, is its own mandala. It is an institute that was founded on the basis of awakening in this lifetime for the benefit of self and others. I'm just aware of how the mandala of CIIS was there at the start for me, at age nineteen, in a way that I had no conscious awareness of, and that I now participate in that mandala as a professor there, teaching students in training to become psychotherapists, to become clinical psychologists.

Eva: It's almost like the future was reaching back toward you as a young adult and calling you toward it.

Willow: Yes. The dreambody of CIIS was present even as I was in my second year at Stanford and completely unaware of it.

Eva: And yet its influence was beginning to permeate and shape you and call you forth into your own journey, your own trajectory, that eventually led you here.

Willow: Do we want to say anything, before we close, returning to your earlier dream, about any links that might be available in your awareness between being the passenger driving the car with your mind, being the rider of the bicycle, leaving Shambhala, and the scream that is heard?

Eva: Yes. There's something about finding one's own unique vehicle for transformation that's arising for me. There are certain pre-prescribed vehicles, whether they're religious or educational institutions or spiritual communities. And sometimes we think that these institutions will be the vehicle that's going to transport us to the next stage in our lives and growth. Yet I think there are all these secret or alternative vehicles that we get to discover. Like that soundproof music room being that incubator for you, that safe holding space. That was its own unique vehicle. And in the dream that I was sharing with you, I didn't feel comfortable in the institution of that particular monastery. I was literally in the dark searching for some other vehicle. I had to trust in my own mind, which is really the essence of so much of the Buddhist teachings: to begin to develop that trust and relationship with seeing how your mind can be a source of guidance, to be aware of the mind that is guiding you.

Willow: I so appreciate hearing what you're saying, and I feel deeply seen and heard in the sourcing, listening to, learning from, and following the secret vehicle of Chinnamunda/Chinnamasta. She is a deity, a dreambody, that I include in my dedication for our book.

Eva: It brings the dedication alive to know more of her story, symbolism, and embodied expression, and I want to go look up her images now.

Willow: There's a wonderful image of her in Miranda Shaw's book, *Buddhist Goddesses of India* (2006). Chinnamasta is in Chapter 20, the severed-headed goddess (pp. 403–417). And also, there is a wonderful image of Chinnamasta depicted in Alana Fairchild's *Kali Oracle: Ferocious Grace and Supreme Protection with the Wild Divine Mother* (2021/2022), card number 20, described in her accompanying guidebook (pp. 120–123).

Eva: Thank you. I want to go back to one thing you said: that you thought initially that this chapter would have some kind of resolve to it. I'm appreciating that this scream and the expression of it are very much alive and open-ended at this time in your life. And I think as a woman, as long as we're awake and aware in this world, I would hope that the scream would be alive.

There needs to be space for that emotional truth, whether it's sorrow or outrage or grief for the suffering of our planet, the pain humans inflict on one another and the more-than-human world. But we have so few constructive ways to conduct that energy. It's an inquiry that feels very alive for me right now. On occasion, I've intentionally shattered a ceramic vessel, and it can be a physical and energetic version of a scream. The ceramic imploding and shattering gets to be that energetic dispersal.

Willow: I love that. I am resonating with the image and experience of you and Adam together shattering a vessel—at the closing of your wedding ceremony—that was later to become the kintsugi vessel, through the weaving of gold into its brokenness. I remember you and Adam put the vessel in a burlap bag and shattered it together at the close of your wedding, as a demonstration of the brokenness of this life that is ever in need of healing and repair.

Eva: That was an evolution of a tradition of breaking the glass at the end of a Jewish wedding, which has many interpretations. We didn't want to just leave things shattered. We presented a kintsugi that we made previously together, as a metaphor of how it's our work, individually and as a couple, to do what we can to heal the brokenness of our world. I was all for our evolution of this tradition, having a strong affinity to the art of kintsugi.

Willow: That's the Japanese tradition of repairing ceramics with gold, yes?

Eva: Yes. And in the repair, highlighting the fissures and the fractures through gold veins so that the vessel becomes even more beautiful. The brokenness becomes part of the wholeness.

Willow: Beautiful. Shall we end here? Thank you dear.

Notes

1 *Shambhala* has many meanings, definitions, interpretations, and associations. It is a mythological spiritual kingdom in Tibetan Buddhism. It is also the name of a lineage of meditation centers founded by Chögyam Trungpa Rinpoche in the West.

2 This expression "from a scream to a dream" was communicated to me by Ofra Eshel (personal communication, January 4, 2024) and Michael Eigen (personal communication, 2023); both linked to the dreamwork of psychoanalyst Wilfred Bion. Several authors invoke this transformation of F in O [*Faith in O*] or T in O [*Transformation in O*] as "screaming into dreaming" in Bloch and Daws (2015).

3 Buddhism is expressed through multiple *vehicles*, or teaching approaches, the *Hinayana* (or beginning vehicle), the *Mahayana* (or vehicle of the middle way), the *Vajrayana* (or ultimate vehicle), and their combined methods and realizations.

4 For a penetrating illumination and transmission of sound-emptiness-sound, see S. Bloch (2010).

5 See Ofra Eshel's (2019) work on the "Vanished Last Scream" for the clinical implications of intuiting/hearing/dreaming a buried soul scream, which is a background presence and catalyst for this chapter.

6 For a felt sense of Kali, see Bloch (2015) and Kempton (2013, pp. 117–146).

7 Our therapeutic reconnection, thirty-three years later, is held in the context of synchronicities (Marlo, 2022), uncanny communications (Eshel, 2016), and the ways in which memories, held as waking dreams, can be the sources of potential new births.

8 Studying with psychoanalyst and musician Michael Eigen, through his online workshop since 2014 and through his online seminars since 2020 and as a participant in this international Eigen mandala, has been a principal conduit of my ongoing learning from Eigen's furthering of psychoanalyst Wilfred Bion's presencing of a double arrow between catastrophe and faith, each implicating the other, as nondual emotional truth.
9 Chinnamunda/Chinnamasta embraces Hinduism and Buddhism and yet she is not bound by either tradition; she transcends traditional notions of religion, invoking, embodying, and transmitting a spirituality that belongs to the realm of the sacred feminine, which is itself beyond name and form even as she takes on infinite names and forms. See Kempton (2013, pp. 259–278). Also see Miranda Shaw's book *Buddhist Goddesses of India* (2006). Chinnamasta is in Chapter 20, the severed headed goddess (pp. 403–417). Also visit https://teahouse.buddhistdoor.net/chinnamunda/

References

Bloch, S. (2010). "Night is a sound": Music of the black sun. In P. W. Ashton & S. Bloch (Eds.), *Music and psyche: Contemporary psychoanalytic explorations* (pp. 193–212). Spring Journal Books.

Bloch, S. (2015). Bion, eigen, and the dreaming of Kali. In S. Bloch & L. Daws (Eds.), *Living moments: On the work of Michael Eigen*. Routledge.

Bloch, S., & Daws, L. (2015). *Living moments: On the work of Michael Eigen*. Routledge.

Eaton, J. (2015). Becoming a welcoming object: Personal notes on Michael Eigen's impact. In S. Bloch & L. Daws (Eds.), *Living moments: On the work of Michael Eigen* (pp. 131–148). Routledge.

Eshel, O. (2016). In search of the absent analyst: Commentary on Janine de Payer's "uncanny communication." *Psychoanalytic Dialogues*, *26*(2), 185–197.

Eshel, O. (2019). The vanished last scream: Winnicott and Bion. *Psychoanalytic Quarterly*, *88*(1), 111–140.

Fairchild, A. (2021/2022). *Kali oracle: Ferocious grace and supreme protection with the wild divine mother*. Blue Angel Publishing.

Fromm, E. (1994). *Escape from freedom*. Macmillan.

Kempton, S. (2013). *Awakening Shakti: The transformative power of the goddesses of yoga*. Sounds True.

Marlo, H. (2022). Experiencing the spiritual psyche: Reflections on synchronicity-informed psychotherapy. *Jung Journal: Culture & Psyche*, *16*(4), 44–69, https://doi.org/10.1080/19342039.2022.2125770

Ogden, T. (2006). *This art of psychoanalysis: Dreaming undreamt dreams and interrupted cries*. Routledge.

Pearson, W. (2021). Reckoning with the spiritual truth of aversive emotions: Evolving unconditional positive regard and discovering the good enough clinician. In W. Pearson & H. Marlo (Eds.), *The spiritual psyche: Mysticism, intersubjectivity, and psychoanalysis* (pp. 118–137). Routledge.

Shaw, M. (2006). *Buddhist goddesses of India*. Princeton University Press.

2

WATCH

Learning from Time

Nested Dreams

Before I present my waking dreamscape, in three nested dreams, I wish to describe what I mean by nested dreams and nested dreaming and how it is both distinct from and consonant with established definitions, which I have come to be aware of through the process of writing this book.

Curtiss Hoffman (2002) proposes based on his own experience of dreaming

> that lucid dreams (or, at least, some lucid dreams) [dreaming when you know you are dreaming] are a special case of "nested" dreams: dreams which are stacked one inside the other like Russian dolls, and in which the dreamer becomes aware of the inner dream within the outer dream. There may be no limit to the number of levels of nesting that can exist … In conclusion, one of the things which the Eastern dream teachings stress is that the goal is not to achieve the ability to dream lucidly [i.e. to dream lucidly in the night while sleeping, but rather to live lucidly in waking life], for the entire realm of waking world experience is considered neither more, nor less real than the dream.

It is deeply compelling to me that this definition of nested dreams offered by Hoffman, an archaeologist and consciousness researcher who is the former chair of the Department of Anthropology at Bridgewater State College in Massachusetts, is consonant with how the term *nested dreams* has also emerged for me experientially (independent of knowing that this term was in existence in the collective). Of particular note, Hoffman's definition already deeply expands the more conventional view of nested dreaming as occurring only within nighttime

DOI: 10.4324/9781003591863-3

dreams. As illustration of this conventional view, Google AI (searched on June 19, 2025) states that

> Nested dreams, also known as dreams within dreams, involve experiencing a dream where you believe you've woken up, only to realize that you are still dreaming. This can involve multiple layers of dreams, with the dreamer believing they've woken up multiple times before truly awakening. These dreams can be vivid and disorienting, blurring the lines between dream and reality.

Whereas the conventional definition of nested dreams relegates the phenomenon of a "dream within a dream within a dream" and "waking up within a dream to find you're in another dream" to nighttime dreaming, I am using the term of *nested dreams* to apply to all phenomena. I am looking at life itself and our interdependence throughout waking and nighttime dreams as a kaleidoscope of nested dreams, consonant with Hoffman's sense of "lucid living" and then taking it a step further. This further step is a radical interdependence of nested dreaming as "lucid living and dying," inclusive of all stages of consciousness, as a field of continuous un/consciousness.

Expanding upon Hoffman's concept of "lucid living," I am invoking the term *nested dreams* to also refer to myriad experiences of synchronicity. And by synchronicity, I mean the uncanny sense that acausal phenomena happen in resonant relationship to one another, often opening the experiencer to a deep sense of interdependence (see Marlo, 2022, for further exposition on synchronicity). I am interested in how synchronicity is ubiquitous; it is never not happening. It's just that we are not always aware of the ubiquity of synchronicity given our limited human perspectives. I am using the term *nested dreams* to invoke the sense of living and dying as a continuous process of synchronicity, dimensions of which remain unconscious even as we awaken to other dimensions.

It is with this view of nested dreaming as a frame for synchronistic living and dying, both in our ongoing awakenings to "dreams within dreams within dreams" and, in our simultaneous beholding of ever further reaches of mystery, that I now turn to a waking dreamscape that opens me to "learning from time."

Waking Dreamscape

Here is my waking dreamscape in three nested waking dreams[1]: being gifted with my grandmother's watch, taking the bodhisattva vow, and getting married.

I remember my Granny Q. This is the name that I called my mother's mother. *Q* was short for Queenie May, as she was named, being born in Canada on the Queen's birthday. I remember my Granny Q wearing her silver watch with diamond chips, adorning her right wrist. She wore it every day. And when she died, my mother passed my Granny Q's watch on to me. I was grateful to receive my Granny Q's watch and to wear it on special occasions in her memory. Across the years, as I joined with the watch and the living memory of my Granny Q that it carries, I began to wear it on a regular basis.

My Granny Q was a special grandparent to me. She was deeply loving, and as an expression of her love, she wrote poems, which she would type out on thin typing paper. Not only that, but also, among the subjects of her poems, she wrote about my beloved childhood cat, Smokey—writings about life as she imagined Smokey's perspective on it. She would leave these original poems on my pillow for me to find.

I can remember traveling on the bus for the first time by myself, at about age six, to visit her at her apartment, a few miles away from my house, in Toronto, Canada, where I was born and where I lived my early childhood. Spending the night in her bedroom, sleeping in her second twin bed, adjacent to her bed, engendered a profound sense of comfort and belonging.

Fast forward to when I took the Mahayana bodhisattva vow at age thirty-seven with my root teacher Khenpo Tsültrim Gyamtso Rinpoche.[2] Taking this bodhisattva vow was a ritualization, formalization, invocation, and embodiment of Rinpoche's acceptance of me as his student. Taking the bodhisattva vow was my embrace of the heart essence transmission of his teaching, of the inseparability of compassion and wisdom, and of my commitment to a nascent and ever-evolving practice, understanding, and integration of his teachings. In taking the Mahayana bodhisattva vow, one vows to always practice compassion. "The Bodhisattva Vow is the aspiration to awaken for the benefit of all beings. Engaging in the journey to awaken so that we can benefit all beings … deeply aligns us with the truth of our interconnectedness with all beings" (personal communication, Lama Palden Drolma, Sukhasiddhi Foundation, September 13, 2024).

The vow is taken with a teacher in which one has great faith. And the vow is taken after completing a series of preliminary practices[3] on the Buddhist path, including prostrations, recitations, and meditations that cultivate dedication and devotion. My friend Don Milani, a student of Chögyam Trungpa Rinpoche, explained when I reached out to him asking how to prepare to take this vow, that it is customary to bring a gift to Rinpoche in a heartfelt gesture of respect, love, and devotion. I would gift Rinpoche with something precious, I thought, something that I would give up, something that I would give away.

I could not think of any material object more precious to me than my Granny Q's watch, imbued as it was with my lifestream, my family lineage, and the deepest of love. These cherished things I presented to Rinpoche, in the symbolic, material form of my Granny Q's watch.

Rinpoche accepted the watch, holding it in his hand, and received it in silent moments. Then he slowly and deliberately said to me, holding it lightly in his palm, "You should keep this, and meditate on the nature of time." With this instruction and invitation, he returned the watch to me, now transformed from an object of family lineage to an object of meditative practice within a spiritual lineage, becoming a dream image.

It was only in choosing to wear this treasured watch on my wedding day, at age fifty-one, that I was able to conjoin the depth of love from my Granny Q, from my mother, and from Rinpoche—and to integrate my evolving family lineage with the heart essence of the Buddhist yogic path—with embrace of my union with my husband.

I remember the photographer, taking photographs of me as a bride just before the wedding ceremony. He pointed out that I was wearing my watch, as if to indicate a lapse of awareness on my part, prompting me to now take it off. I affirmed my conscious choice to wear the watch, keeping it on my wrist, happy to have it memorialized by photo. In this way, the watch became a sign for meditating on appearance–emptiness–appearance (or appearance–emptiness–opening), a transmission of "illusion-like samadhi,"[4] which is a continuous awareness of the dreamlike true nature of all phenomena.

Throughout my wedding ceremony, in the dynamic ground of my awareness, the deepest of links between my maternal lineage, the guru of my own mind, and the guru of relationship were ushered in. In taking this second vow in my life, my marriage vow, I carried the first vow, the bodhisattva vow, in my innermost heart and so began to thread them together. I have been living that dynamic ground in a continuously evolving presence and awareness of commitment to compassion and awakening love, on the conjoined transpersonal and personal levels, ever since.

Rinpoche's death on June 22, 2024, is yet another meditation on this depth of love and the integration of lineages, through a contemplation on the nature of time. He is gone beyond and yet his teaching lives on. This watch, which he tenderly received and released, teaches time's one-pointed arrow—flying in all directions at once and including the still point of the present moment—as a revelation of timelessness. This timelessness is expressed as the simultaneity and contiguity of past, present, and future, in the dependently arisen appearance of time *as* past, present, and future. Thus, orientation to time is one of inhabiting the here and now of not only the present moment but also its inclusion of the presence of "there and then" and the presence of "what may be."

Love itself is, as it has ever been, my one true spiritual path. A dream path. A timeless path that has no beginning and no end.

Day by day, I behold my Granny Q's watch on my wrist, adorned with the tiny diamond chips that glint in the sun. Through the cycles of its winding and unwinding, I touch this emotional truth of love's true nature.

Dream Dialogue: Holding Watch

Eva: Thank you, Willow, for sharing your waking dream of love in so many dimensions. I feel such tenderness in receiving it.

Willow: In the telling of these nested waking dreams, it really brings into relief for me the truth that compassion has both its peaceful and wrathful dimensions, appearances, and expressions. I think about the threading of the seeming opposites to the love and belonging that taking the bodhisattva vow with Rinpoche and entering marital union with Daniel, joined with my maternal lineage through my Granny Q, convey. The telling of these dreams doesn't broadcast or signal or demonstrate the lack of belonging and the loneliness and the searching and isolation and the feeling of the absence of love that all of those communions are an antidote to.

Eva: I was so struck when you said that love has been your dream path. And this path is not all just a lovely dream. It includes loneliness, isolation, disconnection, longing, and fear. I definitely relate to all of that being included in the dream path of love.

Willow: Those are all-inclusive aspects of these three nested waking dreams—the dialectic of disconnection and connection and the illusion of separateness that belies an underlying interdependence.

Eva: The dream is a search for belonging. It appears as a field of disconnection until there are those points of union, whether it's with your teacher or your grandmother or your husband. And that, too, may be a false dichotomy: the appearance of disconnection contrasting with these apex moments of connection. Yet that very dichotomy is part of the tumultuous searching journey for belonging in this lifetime. The dream of searching for love looks different for each person. Longing is nestled in belonging.

Willow: That's beautifully said.

Eva: It reminds me of one of my favorite books from childhood, *The Heart Is a Lonely Hunter,* by Carson McCullers. I've since forgotten much of the content, and yet the title imbues an emotional truth: the heart *is* a lonely hunter as we try to find the people, relationships, and communities that make us feel like we're meant to be here.

Willow: It's striking to me as somebody who has experienced her only marriage at age fifty-one, how there's a sense in which I needed to take great leave of this world of appearances (in order to come back to it with a sense of appearance–emptiness–appearance). I could not find myself in this worldly realm. I have very much been a seeker throughout my life and gravitated to spiritual practice. The paradoxical spiritual sense of belonging—which is a belonging of no one (the sense of touching a realization of no-self) and finding no home—has allowed me to source a sense of connection in this world that allowed me to connect with (my husband) Daniel and forge a relationship with him.

Eva: The relative and the absolute, if those words resonate, are both operating simultaneously, and you don't want to erase one for the other. I spent much of my early twenties too as a seeker, living at a Zen monastery, while my peers were off in the marketplace, finding a partner, settling down, getting married; I have always taken a different, wayward path.

Love was such a huge part of that path, but it didn't necessarily look like a traditional form of love located in one person, and yet I think there was great intimacy in the path that I was traveling.

Willow: I relate to your experience in all of those ways.

Eva: Yes, I think we've been circumambulating a mountain, but at different points. And then finally we caught up and saw each other, side by side, on the path up the mountain.

Willow: ... Spiraling up, down, and around the mountain.

Eva: Yes.

Willow: And the winding and unwinding of the watch feels like such an important dream image that I do practice daily when I put on my Granny Q's watch and notice that time has stopped on its face and that I need to wind it again so that time can continue. There's this sense of limited time and also this sense of endless time and how they interact.

There is, in my present beholding of the watch, this sense of my Granny Q's passing when I was eighteen and Rinpoche's recent death just two months ago, and the awareness of this gift of time to be in relationship with Daniel and never knowing how long our lives and our life together will be and what we will be graced and challenged with. The dream watch reminds me to be in the present even as time is unfolding. And the dream watch also reminds me of the nature of time, in the expression of writing these nested dreams about time's one-pointed arrow flying in all directions. It is this paradox of time being now and yet also unfolding in past, present, and future in both a contiguous way and a synchronous way. And I feel like that's one of the most meaningful teachings embedded in these three nested dreams, these three waking dreams, and the way that Rinpoche's instruction offers an invitation of contemplation, showing me the nested nature of these three waking dreams.

Eva: That was such a powerful moment when you were willing to release the watch, which holds so much significance and connection to your grandmother. I felt so many different emotions when I heard you say that you were about to relinquish the watch. I was a bit stunned because those family heirlooms are irreplaceable and take on a much bigger meaning than the thing itself. And yet the way that he transfixed and transformed the symbol of the watch by offering it back to you also took my breath away.

Willow: ... And holding it first, receiving it first before he gave it back to me. Taking in the gift of my watch, receiving my gesture of letting go and offering and supplication.

Eva: Right. In this object is your ancestral lineage, and now his lineage is attached to it as well. His love is intertwined with your grandmother's love. Incidentally, I spent this last weekend going through family heirlooms at my parents' home, many of which I had never seen before. I really felt into the presence, particularly of my maternal grandmother, in specific items that she had: handkerchiefs that she had embroidered and strings of gray pearls. And I took several of these things, not entirely sure of what my relationship will be to them given that I don't tend to wear pearls out in the world. But I also feel like these objects are imbued with my grandmother's presence, and maybe I will touch the pearls like a mala or Buddhist prayer beads in my hand.

And then I thought of your dream, of what it would be to give those things up, and how it would need to be for something so much bigger than myself. Again, pointing to the absolute dimension of being that we're speaking about. Knowing the object is both an expression of absolute and relative truth simultaneously. I am also imagining when I'm no longer here, what are the things that will have my spirit within them, considering that I am a future ancestor as well. Whether it is my wedding ring or some other object, what will be the things that people will behold and say, "Oh yes, that was my great aunt Eva's." While they are just objects, they are also embodiments of love and memory.

Willow: Absolutely. I'm really touched by your expression of recognition within your own direct experience of what it would be like to give some of those things up and that doing so would have to be something that moved you to a very deep expression of the absolute. And I also hear you affirming with me that the absolute and relative are ever co-emergent—as in your holding your grandmother's gray pearls like a mala. There's the object, the dream object, the dream image. Holding my Granny Q's watch as a dream image is just that: It's the teaching that's now infused in that watch for me and the double entendre of *watch* as object and *watch* as verb. A teaching of watching the watcher. A teaching about how, in addition to letting it go and offering it as a gift, it was equally important to have the watch returned to me and have the watch continue.

[The Zoom call disconnects on Eva's end, and Willow doesn't initially realize it. Then Eva calls Willow on the phone, and they continue recording their conversation through Zoom, which Eva is physically absent from.]

As you were trying to link back on Zoom, I was just articulating the double entendre of *watch* as object and *watch* as verb. And I'm aware of not realizing at first that you disappeared, and then realizing it and having a range of feelings, including, "Oh my God, where did Eva go?

When is she coming back?" And then settling in with a sense of "I don't know what's happening. I don't know where she went, but I can be in touch with her presence, in her absence, and I can wait and see."

Eva: Yes, and in a way the watch's absence and presence together as well: the absence of your grandmother and the presence of your grandmother and seeing Rinpoche, awareness of both departure and return coinciding.

Willow: I was thinking about that particularly in terms of wearing the watch on my wedding day and how the presence of the watch carried an awareness of the inevitability, the eventuality, of absence as well, not as nihilistic forlornness, but as recognition of the grace of the time that we do have.

Eva: Wedding vows really put that front and center. I certainly felt that very much after that rite of passage. The ceremony held the understanding that if we are committing to walk this path together, there may be a point where only one of us is walking the path without the other.

Willow: You felt that in your own marriage ceremony with Adam?

Eva: Yes. I still feel it. He was away for the last ten days, without any cellphone reception; at a certain point we must find a way to carry the relationship within us, even if the person isn't there to talk to. I find this very challenging.

Willow: When you disappeared on the Zoom screen just a moment ago, part of me wanted to bypass your absence and keep talking to you. There was a usefulness in continuing the conversation and a spiritual bypass at the same time. Part of me was staying in connection with you, but I was doing so in a way that I wasn't actually taking in the disjuncture of our dis/connection.

Eva: Yes. And oftentimes in life we're forced to do so when someone we love isn't here to have the dialogue in person, but we still continue talking to them or relating to them. Maybe it's not in language but in feeling into their presence and simultaneously their absence. The watch is part of that dialogue for you, I imagine.

Willow: Very much so. I mean, Granny Q has been gone for thirty-six years now, and Rinpoche has been gone for just two months, and yet the last time I physically saw him was sixteen years ago. So, there were sixteen years that he was living in Nepal that I didn't have an audience with him, didn't have interviews with him, but very much carried him on the inner spiritual plane in terms of working with his teachings, which I continue to do now that he's gone beyond.

Eva: It's so interesting because as you're sharing this, a dream I had very early this morning before waking is rising back up for me. I knew that we would be discussing this dream today, about your watch and about your taking the bodhisattva vow. And so I wonder if there's any synchronicity in that I haven't had many dreams of my first Zen Buddhist teacher. I have not been in touch with him for probably two decades. *In the dream, I was bobbing up and down in the swells of the ocean, and these big waves were crashing over me, and I said something to the extent that I didn't like how it felt to have the waves crashing over my head. And then I looked up and my Zen Buddhist teacher rose up out of the waves in his priest robes and said that he would be glad to take me back home. I said, "It's quite late at night. Do you have time?" And he said, "Oh, I always have time to take you home."*

There was this vitality and joy, even as my last memories of him were that he was more fragile and in his aging process, but in the dream, he seemed very playful, spontaneously arising out of the waves. And he took me back to my childhood home. It's so interesting to have had that dream in the hours leading up to this conversation, in which I knew we would be talking about your teacher.

Willow: That's such a powerful sentence: "I always have time to take you home."

Eva: Yes. And I really felt the relief in that because I didn't like feeling pushed about by the waves. I was doing my best, but I was actually quite relieved that he was going to bring me to *terra firma*. There's a lot of sweetness in my relationship with my teacher that continues to exist in dreams, even though I haven't been in touch with him for so many years.

Willow: Beautiful. I'm also aware at this moment that it can seem like, in our conversation, the hardest thing to do is to surrender to the absolute, but I feel like it's equally hard to surrender to the relative. And that both truths are what allow for each recognition of their co-emergence. I feel like growing into those two truths allowed me to open to the capacity to marry Daniel—to grow into the capacity to be here, as just me, loving him, in our life together. And that being able to embrace the absolute, or what we could call the emptiness dimension of appearances, or forms, is certainly what partnered me in allowing that dream of marrying Daniel to arise, now allowing this dream of marriage to be lived.

And I am struck in your sharing of this dream this morning that there's something about bobbing in the ocean. Even if you're going to get struck by the waves. That bobbing around sometimes can feel more at home than terra firma, and that it requires a kind of spiritual bravery and risk-taking to be here fully, just as we are, with all of our radiance and all of our imperfections and limitations, and to allow a real love that's a day-to-day love, which is different than the real love of a spiritual teacher who you see once every so often.

And they're both forms of love. But I think, as we've expressed in Chapter 9, Devotion: Learning from Nondual Love, for me anyway, the first overture of nondual love was learning from spiritual teachers. And for me too, all along the way, I've not been a stranger to intimate love, but that this intimate love with Daniel, my husband, is a new form of showing up with the inevitability of loss, of disappearance, as you brought to the fore in your Zoom disappearance. Loving Daniel is a further daily teaching and practice of awakening nondual love.

Eva: The price of loving deeply is experiencing grief. The two are inseparable, and I often wrestle against that, in wishing that I could love deeply without the fear or reality of loss and yet that is the contract that is signed without consent: If we love in this lifetime, there's this implicit contract that we will also grieve what we have loved.

Willow: And that's the real dream.

Eva: Can you say more about what you mean by that?

Willow: I found myself writing in *The Spiritual Psyche* (Pearson & Marlo, 2021), "dreaming is as real as it gets," meaning that dreaming this waking life, just as dreaming our nighttime dreams, is what we started this conversation with. Namely, we dream apparent opposites, the light and the dark, and the connections and the disconnections; dreaming is all the more real because it touches this thing that we're also circumambulating, as you said, which is this presence that doesn't exclude loss and yet does transcend time. Illusion-like samadhi and cherishment of the real,[5] in the sense that dreaming is as real as it gets, are not two. There is a nondual simultaneity of waking up *from* the illusory nature of being and, in the same breath, waking up *to* cherishment of the luminosity (the illusion as it shines) of this life.

Eva: Yes. Thank you.

Willow: Is there any last note that you wanted to sound before we end?

Eva: Just my gratitude. I feel really moved. I know in painting that a series of something that's in threes is a triptych, but that doesn't quite feel like the word I'm searching for. There's a sequence in each of these pieces, these thirds that culminate in a really beautiful meditation on loving in this life, the watch being the symbol that carries through each of the parts. I really feel how it is the dream image in this waking dream.

Willow: Thank you, dear Eva.

Notes

1 This illustration of "nested dreams" is one of extending and participating in the ever-present Great Seal of the oneiric field (in the sense of Mahamudra). The concept and living of *nested dreams* is a psychotherapeutic and spiritual practice—an affirmative recognition of and response to Edgar Allan Poe's (1850) poem "A Dream Within A Dream" that wonders, "Is all that we see and seem but a dream within a dream?" (see https://www.poetryfoundation.org/poems/52829/a-dream-within-a-dream). The concept and living of *nested dreams* is an extension of and distinction to Civitarese's sense that in *transformations of hallucinosis* one awakens from the hallucination, and this waking from union-distinction (to reverse Eigen's term of distinction-union) is what allows, in part, for the intersubjective transformation. While in agreement, to take this sense further, I would add that we awaken *to another nested dream within a dream*. In other words, illusion-like samadhi may become a continuous rhythm of *transformations in dreaming* (see Ferro, 2015) and *transformations in hallucinosis*. (See Civitarese, 2015). *Nested dreaming*, and by application *nested frames* in psychoanalytic psychotherapeutic practice, is a realization of the continuous nature of dreaming and thus of the un/conscious.

2 *Mahayana* can be translated as Buddhism of the "middle way." One way of understanding this "middle way," as I practice it, is that Mahayana Buddhism is a lived practice and recognition of Self/no-self.

3 See Sukhasiddhi Foundation's overview of depth practice by Lama Döndrup for a sense of this preliminary path and its relationship to the whole: https://www.sukhasiddhi.org/depth-practice-program

4 See Khenpo Tsültrim Gyamtso (2010), https://tricycle.org/magazine/path-faith-and-path-reasoning/, and https://ktgrinpoche.org/songs/verses-samadhi-illusion-texts-middle-way

5 See Lionessroars.org/music/caesuras-cry to hear a song entitled "Cherishing the Real" dedicated to my husband Daniel, one of a fourteen-song cycle—the album is entitled *Caesura's Cry*—about beholding love in its wisdom, compassion, and vision. The song can also be heard on most downloadable and streaming platforms, such as Apple Music, SoundCloud, and Spotify, under *Caesura's Cry* by Willow Pearson Trimbach.

References

Civitarese, G. (2015). Transformations in hallucinosis and the receptivity of the analyst. *The International Journal of Psychoanalysis*, *96*(4), 1091–1116. https://doi.org/10.1111/1745-8315.12242

Ferro, A. (2015). *Torments of the soul: Psychoanalytic transformations in dreaming and narration*. Routledge.

Hoffman, C. (2002). Lucid dreams, nested dreams. *Evolution of the Dream Movement, Dream Network, 21*(4). https://dreamnetworkjournal.com/bcpoy5zfldnd/lucid-dreams-nested-dreams

Khenpo, T. G. (2010). The path of faith and the path of reasoning: Dissecting devotion. *Tricycle* (Spring). https://tricycle.org/magazine/path-faith-and-path-reasoning/

Marlo, H. (2022). Experiencing the spiritual psyche: Reflections on synchronicity-informed psychotherapy. *Jung Journal: Culture & Psyche*, *16*(4), 44–69, https://doi.org/10.1080/19342039.2022.2125770

Pearson, W., & Marlo, H. (Eds.). (2021). *The spiritual psyche in psychotherapy*. Routledge.

Poe, E. A. (1850). A dream within a dream. In R. W. Griswold (Ed.), *The works of the late Edgar Allan Poe*. J. S. Redfield. Public Domain.

3

SONG

Learning from Singing—Guru Bodhichitta

Here, in this chapter, "Song: Learning from Singing—Guru Bodhichitta," the dream translates itself into music. As we share the dream song, "Guru Bodhichitta," from Willow's original music catalogue as "The Watermoons," we learn from the innermost teaching of primordial wisdom and compassion, aware of its own nature. Through the ultimate teacher, *Awakened Heart* (Almaas, 2023a, 2023b), as bodhichitta can be translated, the singer as dreamer begins to hear her own voice and so, too, her life-affirming link to the heart of the cosmos. We illustrate the relationship between singing and dreaming, as the conjoined external and internal voices of the soul echoing inside and outside at once. Through the resonant emotional truth of the lyrics set to music, the practice and fruition of meditation is sung into being as a guide to dreaming.

Guru Bodhichitta[1]

music by Eric Ramstad, lyrics by The Watermoons
recorded on The Watermoons' first album, *Red Boat*

Still your mind, like a river that runs through
Still your mind, like a river that runs true
Look behind and beneath the riverbed
There you'll find all the things that need be said

Guru Bodhichitta Namami
Guru Bodhichitta Namami

Still your mind, in the light that comes through you
There you'll find the love you always knew

DOI: 10.4324/9781003591863-4

Everyone here is waking in the Now
Listen close, let the Guru show you how

Guru Bodhichitta Namami
Guru Bodhichitta Namami

May all beings be free of suffering
May all beings live in equality

Like a dream ... when you know you are dreaming

Guru Bodhichitta Namami
Guru Bodhichitta Namami

Guru Bodhichitta Namami
Guru Bodhichitta Namami

Guru Bodhichitta Namami
Guru Bodhichitta Namami

Guru Bodhichitta Namami
Guru Bodhichitta Namami

Willow: "Guru Bodhichitta" is my favorite song on *Red Boat* (The Watermoons, 2012), an album that I co-wrote with my dear friend and dharma brother Eric Ramstad, in part because of its great simplicity and the insistence on reverent repetition. The song stems from and originates as an homage to the definitive Guru, Bodhichitta.

Bodhichitta can be defined as the inseparability of wisdom and compassion, and bodhichitta can be expressed as *Awakened Heart*, arising from a desire to be of benefit to oneself and others. The song, itself a form of dreaming,[2] a conduit of emotional truth, is simply an unfolding, an ever-deepening recognition, of just that definition and expression: that life itself can be understood and lived as an homage to the great, unsurpassable Guru Bodhichitta—the spiritual teacher that is Awakened Heart.[3]

The song's repetitive refrain is "Guru Bodhichitta Namami." The word *Namami* is an invocation of homage. The dreamer sings, in essence, "I pay homage to the ultimate Guru." On one level, I am singing to Mahasiddha Khenpo Tsültrim Gyamtso Rinpoche, my root teacher, who is inseparable from all my teachers and who shines as all appearances, without a single one left out. This is on the outer level. On a deeper level, I am singing from the guru of my own mind, inseparable from all appearances and their inherent dreamlike nature. This is on the inner level. And, on another level of depth, I am singing from within the guru of relationship—the living emotional truths of interpersonal connections and their inherent dreamlike nature that are, in meaningful respects, quite private from others. This is on a secret level.

And on the innermost level of the song, lies the nondual union of all levels of awareness—this great seal of awareness and expression as dreaming Guru Bodhichitta.

This dream teaching about paying homage to the ultimate Guru came in the form of a song, inseparable from communion of the heart. At its essence, the dream song teaches me the emotional truth of authentic voice through the composition, the emotional truth of singing my soul's recognition of the ultimate spiritual teacher. It teaches me the emotional truth of hearing my own voice and recognizing my own spiritual authority. It teaches me about touching and being present to my own emotional truth, as a direct, unmediated realization, born through meaningful relationship to my teacher, Rinpoche, and to my dharma brother, Eric, cowriter of the song.

The dreamer sings,

Still your mind, like a river that runs through
Still your mind, like a river that runs true
Look behind and beneath the riverbed,
There you'll find all the things that need be said

In this verse, the petitioner, the composer, the singer, the aspirant, and the seeker, has a deep question about right speech. And there is guidance in this verse about that, which I will unfold here.

"Still your mind." This is the basic instruction of calm abiding, which is the first basis of meditation practice in the Tibetan Buddhist tradition. This first basis of meditation is referred to in Buddhism as *shamatha.* "Still your mind like a river that runs through." These opening lyrics present a paradox. On the one hand we're stilling our mind because the gushing river, the torrent of thoughts that we identify with, needs to come into calmness, into peaceful abiding. But nondual recognition is right there at the onset of the song in that very line. As the whole line sings, "Still your mind like the river that runs through." Your mind *is* that stillness *inseparable from the river*, that stream of thought that runs through you. So contained in the song, right within that very first calm-abiding (shamatha) instruction, is *mahamudra*, a meditation practice that can be translated in short as "great [hand] seal" of all phenomena or as the "great embrace,"[4] with not a single thing left out, shining as Guru Bodhichitta (Rinpoche, 2016; Kyabgon, 2004, 2015; Harding, 2013; Rinpoche, 2003).

The second line of the dream song is "Still your mind, like a river that runs true." So this expression deepens, echoes, and penetrates that nondual clarity, right within the first principle of calm abiding, of stillness, of taking your seat, of finding your feet.

The next line of Guru Bodhichitta is "Look behind and beneath the riverbed." In this line, "Look behind and beneath the riverbed" the song exhorts us to look for what is essential. Look for that which is core. The song entreats, don't be simply swept or carried along by first thoughts, impulsiveness. Here, there is a call to discriminating wisdom. Then, there is a call to look behind and beneath the riverbed of discursive mind. This is a call to ethical conduct through right speech. Also, at once, there is play and laughter here; there is no "behind," no "beneath." There is nothing there, in the sense of there being no permanent existence, no truly separate existence. There is only the looking, the emptiness, the inseparability. And, also, at once, not even the looking is truly existent; when you look directly at the looking, it dissolves. And, too, this looking shines forth! Emptiness opens! This too is an expression and embodiment of mahamudra, great hand seal, great embrace, as taught by Guru Bodhichitta.

I want to pause here, Eva, and check in and see how you're doing. How are you relating to my commentary on the dream song?

Eva: It's very moving to me. Shall I share what's arising as I'm listening?

Willow: Absolutely.

Eva: As I'm receiving the dream song, which in and of itself is a beautiful phrase and concept, I'm feeling moved in response to the night that I just woke up from, which actually didn't involve a lot of sleep. I couldn't sleep because a very important teacher in my life just entered hospice. I learned last night that she was actively dying, and it was almost like my soul was keeping vigil over her. I couldn't fully surrender. I was very awake to the fact that one of my greatest teachers of the creative spirit—whom I consider a mystic philosopher—is exiting this realm. I was really wrestling in the night with the finiteness of our relationship ending.

As I feel into what you're speaking to here, to the absolute nature of it, I touch the truth that the guru, the teacher, exists within me as well. And so as I'm receiving this commentary on the dream song, it feels like a mirror of my sleepless night. My soul was really tossing and turning with what it means to lose the in-person contact and the back-and-forth dialogue with someone who has known me my whole life and is a guru in a certain way. Yet I also feel like I've internalized her voice; it's a matter of really trusting that it's there, that even as her physical form is dissolving and her consciousness is departing, that I will have the teacher always abiding within me.

And I am living the lines about the paradox of the stillness of the mind and the fluidity of the river and trying to find the truth within that paradox. I've been feeling that as a part of me tries to find calm abiding, recognizing the impermanence of all life, another part feels into a torrent of anguish and grief. But then trying to access the fundamental okayness with what is happening as well. So Guru Bodhichitta is really speaking to me in light of the night that I've just experienced.

Willow: Thank you so much for invoking and sharing the presence of this tossing and turning on the level of soul that you're experiencing with your dear friend and teacher.

Eva: Thank you. It feels very synchronistic to revisit this dream song at this moment in time.

Willow: Shall I continue with the dream-song commentary and we'll see what else comes forward?

Eva: Yes.

Willow: The next line sings, "There you'll find all the things that need be said." So there's play and laughter that echoes here as well. This lyric is pointing out that there's nothing to find. And finding that is a great joy. It's a paradoxical exhortation to silence: there's nothing to find. There's nothing there. What could possibly need to be said? Ultimately there is no riverbed. No unchanging ground. So, in this way, this verse is about the wisdom of silence. Of containment. Of right speech as no speech. And, once again paradoxically, the lyrics are (themselves an embodiment of right speech as song), at once, about the words that this situation calls for. In this way, simply by practicing meditation and so joining with mahamudra, by joining calm abiding with the beginning movement toward insight, the singer opens into the nature of mind that is naturally present.

That clarity is invoked with the line "look behind and beneath the riverbed." So the first two lines are about calm abiding, or shamatha practice; and the third line is about insight, or vipassana practice; and the last line is about conduct, about ethics, in the form of right speech. The last line sings, "There you'll find all the things that need be said." The song teaches the listener to join stillness, calm abiding, with insight, to recognize the nature of mind; the song teaches that in joining with Guru Bodhichitta, the embodiment of wisdom and compassion, the listener will find the oars for the red boat: living passionately with full expression, that choiceful capability to be silent, to not speak, and, equally, to spontaneously meet the moment with their expressive mark of existence.

Then the chorus …

Guru Bodhichitta Namami
Guru Bodhichitta Namami
Guru Bodhichitta Namami

Let me pause here, Eva, and see if there's anything you're called to speak.

Eva: I'm simply feeling the grace of compassion in this process of navigating the river. And how turbulent it can often feel. That calm abiding often doesn't feel easily accessed, but that's where compassion surrounds us in the process and can lead to that source of balance, that source of stillness. Often that doesn't happen without tumult, without fluctuation, without the movement of the mind in all its confusion.

That's such a beautiful metaphor of the listener finding the oars of the boat. This conjures the song from my childhood: "Row, row, row your boat, gently down the stream. Merrily, merrily, merrily life is but a dream." It can feel so turbulent and challenging to be rowing down the stream, but then to also hold in mind that it is also but a dream.

Willow: So beautifully said.

Eva: Thank you. What you wrote, about the red boat, is really such a poignant image.

Willow: Shall we take that image and go further?

Eva: Sure.

Willow: All of this is homage to the unsurpassable Guru of Bodhichitta, the indivisible union of wisdom and compassion. The dream song carries the understanding that these very instructions of meditation come from the kindness of our teachers with their devotion to truth. These instructions point out and are themselves the nature of a dream. Their understanding—that if you too can practice meditation, in meditation and post-meditation, you can be of even greater benefit to others, including yourself—is celebrated here.

So when Milarepa sings that "those who inspire others to take up this call/Their kindness stretches far too great to tell," that is exactly the case (personal communication, Lama Palden Drolma, Sukhasiddhi Foundation, 2012). Every teacher and therapist who has inspired us to work with and open our mind and heart has touched us with bodhichitta. They have demonstrated the nature of a bodhisattva, in that commitment, in that service. Those teachers who have practiced and studied and coalesced a dharma center, an institute, a foundation, a studio, a classroom, a consulting room, in order to offer us instruction in meditation and psychotherapy—the living arts, the healing arts—offer us a great gift.

Those teachers who have accomplished *mahamudra* in view (or outlook), meditation, conduct, and fruition inseparable are the true masters we pay the deepest homage to, praying that they will remain in this world to guide wandering beings such as ourselves, through their transmission, their blessing, their teaching, their enlightened activity, their supreme example. We pray that we will be just like them down the line, in our own unique way, one practice session and post-meditation experience at a time. We discover that we are always already inseparable from the nature of mind. We discover our own personal expression of dharma, of truth, just as it is, in this very moment, and in this unique offering we discover how our mind is inseparable from the Guru, Bodhichitta. We are dreaming Guru Bodhichitta, just as Guru Bodhichitta is dreaming us.

The next verse sings,

Still your mind in the light that comes through you
There you'll find the love you always knew
Everyone here is waking in the now
Listen close, let the guru show you how

Here, again, the song is returning our attention to the first principle in mahamudra meditation, to calm abiding, to shamatha. "Still your mind in the light that comes through you."

There is something in this line about not getting carried away in the ecstasy, the bliss, at those times when bliss shows its face as the *preferred* radiance. Not the all-pervading radiance of genuine equality but the preferred radiance of relative reality where we source inspiration, and goodness, and beauty. Still your mind. Right within that stillness, let go. Right within that passion for this life, find the emptiness within that appearance. Having recognized all appearances as emptiness, touch the emptiness within that appearance, seeing that emptiness is also empty of being empty.

"Still your mind in the light that comes through you / There you'll find the love you always knew." So we have sought out, we have been touched by, and we have been inspired by and given our devotion to the Guru, as an external teacher, or a commitment to working with a therapist, because we thought that they possessed something that we did not possess. And on a certain level that is quite true, that is the case. Our beloved teachers and therapists possess a certain understanding that we do not yet recognize in ourselves. But when, in accordance with our teacher's blessing, our therapist's practice, we join with our teacher's mindstream, taking up a practice of meditation or psychotherapy, we awaken to the nature of mind, as every teacher on the path has ever shown us, continuously out of their great kindness. This is none other than who we've always been, what we've always known, what we've never been separate from, what we're not separate from now nor will we ever be. Even now, as we read these words. Even if we forget this, that it is the indestructible truth. We are dreaming Guru Bodhichitta.

Eva: I feel tearful hearing this because I think that this is the realization that I was tossing and turning with in the night. It is this inseparability between teacher and student—that there can be a golden shadow that we project onto our teachers, that they hold certain capacities that we don't yet have. But the most compelling teachers hold a mirror and show us the ways in which we possess those same qualities. Perhaps we need to grow further into those qualities.

My teacher who is in the process of dying right now selected her students because she saw within them certain qualities that could be nurtured; the seeds were already there, and she was quite intentional in choosing who she taught and mentored. This is a parting gift: that these qualities don't just exist within her and leave with her. But as you said that any beloved teacher or therapist helps us recognize these qualities within ourselves.

Willow: Absolutely.

Eva: It's like they light this flame within us, perhaps what we refer to as Bodhichitta; they continue to light it in the next candle, and then we light it in the next candle, and it just becomes this luminous source that continues to be passed through the lineage.

Willow: Beautifully said. Yes. So this continues very much in that sense. Are you okay for me to read three more pages of commentary, to see where it takes us?

Eva: Yes.

Willow: Okay. "There you'll find the love you always knew." You were right to recognize, the song teaches, the awakened mind of your Guru, in second person, in the transmission of their pure presence, and in third person, through their enlightened activities of building dharma centers and institutes and foundations and nunneries and studios and consulting rooms and classrooms and publishing dharma texts and recording audio files and mentoring translators and providing teaching environments and therapy sessions and classes and retreats and intensives and practice weeks and such. The Guru is teaching you from awakened mind in the first person. And not only that, but also your awakened mind is indivisible from the third person, the environment, the world that we inhabit that inhabits us.

"Everyone here is waking in the now." Everyone, whether they have taken up a spiritual practice in a self-aware way or not, is on the path of this life, and life wakes us up if we're paying attention. It's impossible not to notice this on some level because we all come into this existence taking on a body, and we all have to release the body when we leave. None of us will escape the letting go of loved ones who cross the unknown sea before our time. None of us will escape the awareness that others will cross the unknown sea after our time. And we all seek ways to work with this truth, this dharma, this dream. So, however quickly or slowly we might see progress in ourselves and others, the dreamer is singing, we can rest assured that we are all awakening together, moment by moment, in the now (Almaas, 2014).

Last line of this stanza, "Listen close, let the Guru show you how." Again the exhortation to the yoga of listening. *Nada yoga* is the yoga of sound. Listen. In the balance of silence and expression, to return to the inquiry of right speech, the first principle is to listen. And, of course, that in and of itself is inseparable from that which one listens to. "Listen close." Listen to the innermost. Find ways to quiet all the other layers of cacophonous sound that clamor for your attention and turn that attention inward. "Listen close. Let the guru show you how." On the levels of outer (external teacher), inner (your own mind), secret (your relationships), and innermost (the sacred union of these), and their ultimate equality, do find a way to go within. Be so deeply acquainted with the innermost that you are inseparable from that, which is the union of your mind with the Guru, Bodhichitta. In the land of equality, this is of supreme importance.

May all beings be free of suffering
May all beings live in equality

Like a dream ... when you know you are dreaming

Guru Bodhichitta Namami
Guru Bodhichitta Namami
Guru Bodhichitta Namami

The song closes with a prayer. "*May all beings be free of suffering. May all beings live in equality. Like a dream ... when you know you are dreaming.*" This prayer is a direct teaching from Khenpo Tsültrim Gyamtso Rinpoche, which now arises in my own mindstream, in my own heart, in my own voice, through the dream song. The prayer, the mind training, transmits that all appearances—all phenomena, all sounds, all senses, all thoughts—are like a dream, when you know you are dreaming.

As Guru Bodhichitta teaches, both songs and dreams are conduits and transmissions of emotional truth, written in sound–emptiness–sound (or sound echoing as emptiness opening), conceived in clarity–emptiness–thought (or thought illuminated as emptiness opening), experienced as bliss–emptiness–feeling (or feeling experienced as opening into bliss) and manifest as appearance–emptiness–appearance (or appearance shining as emptiness opening).[5] Songs and art and dreams are expressions of the soul in its intimate knowability and its abiding mystery at once.

Is there anything, Eva, you want to add here or respond to here?

Eva: I am very moved by the way you're able to express through language that which is ephemeral, like a bubble, all that dissolves and the emptiness of reality when you realize, as you said, all phenomena and all sounds, all senses, all thoughts are like a dream and that we can bring our awareness to this, which has a flavor of melancholy, that we can't really hold on to anything. But then also as you later say, in this emptiness, bliss can arise as well. And also beauty through song and art and dreams.

Willow: Thank you. So to close…

If no other mantra, if no other prayer, if no other teaching, return to this one:

Guru Bodhichitta Namami

I pay homage to the Guru of the inseparability of wisdom and compassion on the outer, the inner, the secret, and the innermost levels of dreaming the great teacher, Awakened Heart.

Dreaming Lost and Found

Willow: Deeply listening to Guru Bodhichitta—the expression conducted through my voice and the poetry communicated by the lyrics—has shown me that the Awakened Heart of love is the teacher, not the teacher as an individual. And the dream is the conduit of that love that transcends person, place, time, or situation. As simple a revelation as this may be, it's been a thirty-year process for me to understand, to define, and to live this dream path of nondual love—the essential embrace of Guru Bodhichitta. Coming home to this simple revelation oddly then allows me to hold each of the people who have been my teachers with more acceptance and appreciative regard, indeed, to hold them as sacred mirrors to my own embodiment of ensouled divinity. As conduits of nondual love, each of us is free to be more fully human in our individuality and uniqueness—not divorced from the confluence and entanglement of our wisdom and our confusion.

Eva: What a gift, Willow. Thank you so much. I really needed to hear this. I've been in a state of turmoil for how to reconcile the living, breathing relationship that I've had with my teacher and what it means for her soul and consciousness to depart, for her body to not be here. And she's such an embodied person as a dancer, which was her life's work, but she was so much more than that; she was a teacher of poetry and philosophy and mysticism.

And so this is so helpful for me to recognize that she is within me; I am within her. It's just inseparable. That she is, as you said, a conduit of nondual love and certainly would want me to continue to express my own sensitivities, which she really saw in me from a very young age and helped to cultivate those sensitivities in a way that I really don't think in the broader culture would have been seen or nurtured. I love how you end with the confluence and entanglement of our wisdom and our confusion because it's not purely one or the other. They exist simultaneously. And it makes me feel more okay with my confusion, even as I feel into wisdom, because, at least last night, I was feeling like I shouldn't be feeling this much confusion or anguish.

Actually, there's space for that, too. There's room for that messiness and that actually contributes to the wisdom rather than it needing to be divorced from it. We enfold back again into our own humanity, recognizing how fragile we are, how resilient we are, how unsure we are, how knowing we are.

Willow: So well said.

Eva: I'm left with feeling more compassion for the vulnerability of living the paradox of the calm abiding, that stillness of the riverbed, with the fluctuations of this life that continues to move through in mysterious and sometimes treacherous, sometimes blissful ways.

Willow: Yes.

Eva: But none of it is wrong. The spiritual path doesn't look one way or there's no one way to be a spiritual being. It's not simply calm abiding at all times.

Willow: Right. That's a tool to help us work with ourselves, but that's not the display that's always on display.

Eva: Yes. Rather than experiencing judgment or shame when I can't access calm abiding, instead, I can include the confusion and turbulence; awareness can show up and say, all right, this too is part of mind. This too is part of living in a body that has a porous heart.

Willow: And thank God for that.

Notes

1 Hear song "Guru Bodhichitta" at www.lionessroars.org/music/redboat. See "Guru Bodhichitta" performed live at https://youtu.be/iTr1rXcTKko. You can also hear "Guru Bodhichitta" on streaming and downloadable music services such as iTunes, Spotify,

SoundCloud, Pandora, Deezer, and Amazon Music, under artists *The Watermoons* (Willow Pearson and Eric Ramstad).

2 See Bloch (2024).

3 In this way, Guru Bodhichitta is a contemporary song of realization in the Tibetan Buddhist tradition of the doha. For traditional songs of realization, see Brunnhölzl (2019, 2021) and Heruka (2016).

4 For a translation of Mahamudra from "great seal" to "great embrace," see Epstein (2015).

5 For a penetrating illumination and transmission of "creative emptiness" as the deity Kali (referenced in Chapter 1), the union of aural sound–emptiness–sound, visual appearance–emptiness–appearance, mental clarity–emptiness–thought, and bliss–emptiness–feeling, see Bloch (2015).

References

Almaas, A. H. (2014). *Runaway realization: Living a life of ceaseless discovery*. Shambhala.

Almaas, A. H. (2023a). *Love unveiled: Discovering the essence of the awakened heart*. Shambhala.

Almaas, A. H. (2023b). *Nondual love: Awakening to the loving nature of reality*. Shambhala.

Bloch, S. (2015). Bion, Eigen, and the dreaming of Kali. In S. Bloch & L. Daws (Eds.), *Living moments: On the work of Michel Eigen* (pp. 3–19). Routledge.

Bloch, S. (2024). Music as dreaming. In K. Cohen & L. Daws (Eds.), *Primary process impacts and dreaming the undreamable object in the work of Michael Eigen: Becoming the welcoming object*. Routledge.

Brunnhölzl, K. (2019). *Luminous melodies: Essential dohas of Indian Mahamudra*. Wisdom Publications.

Brunnhölzl, K. (2021). *Milarepa's Kungfu: Mahamudra in his songs of realization*. Wisdom Publications.

Epstein, M. (2015). Distinction-union: A Buddhist reflection on the great embrace. In S. Bloch & L. Daws (Eds.), *Living moments: On the work of Michael Eigen* (pp. 21–31). Routledge.

Rinpoche, K. T. G. (2016). *Progressive stages of meditation on emptiness: Experiential training in meditation, reflection and insight* (L. S. Hookham, Trans.; 3rd ed.). Shrimala Trust.

Harding, S. (2013). *Machik's complete explanation: Clarifying the meaning of Chöd*. Snow Lion Publications.

Heruka, T. (2016). *The hundred thousand songs of Milarepa: A new translation* (C. Stagg, Trans., under the guidance of D. Ponlop Rinpoche). Shambhala.

Kyabgon, T. (2004). *Mind at ease: Self-liberation through Mahamudra meditation*. Shambhala.

Kyabgon, T. (2015). *Moonbeams of Mahamudra: The classic meditation manual*. Shogam.

Rinpoche, D. P. (2003). *Wild awakening: The heart of Mahamudra & Dzogchen*. Shambhala.

4

ALCHEMY OF SOUL

Learning from Creativity and the Unconscious

In this chapter, we explore the interconnectedness of creativity and dreaming through the lens of Jungian depth psychology, focusing on personal experiences and reflections, specifically in Eva's young adult life. This journey of integrating her artistic and academic selves focuses on the role of dreams as a conduit for accessing the unconscious. Artmaking, as an extension of her dream life, allowed her to engage with the unconscious through symbols and imagery.

Using a paper she wrote at Stanford as the launching point, our dialogue emphasizes the importance of honoring the "nondual un/conscious," where creative practice becomes a spiritual path toward individuation. Here, we show how dreams, particularly "creativity dreams," can empower and connect individuals to archetypal energies, fostering a deeper relationship with soul and spirit. By embracing the mystery of the creative process, we allow it to transform and inform both waking and dream life, ultimately leading to a more integrated and fulfilling existence.

Eva: For this dialogue, I wish to invite my younger self into the conversation. When I was twenty years old I was fortunate to study with Dr. Douglas Daher, a Jungian analyst, an outlier in Stanford's Department of Psychology, which was much more behaviorally oriented. For our final paper, Dr. Daher asked us to apply our learnings in Jungian depth psychology to our own dream life. It was the first time in my academic career in which my inner life was invited to be the subject of inquiry. The paper I wrote explores the tension I experienced at that time between my artist self and my academic self, among other polarities, and a deep yearning to uphold my intuition in an environment that often privileged rationality.

Certain themes began to emerge in my dreams then that still show their face today: my courtship—sometimes celebratory, sometimes fraught,

DOI: 10.4324/9781003591863-5

sometimes distant or neglectful—with my inner creative life. Soul has always found a way of revealing in my dreams the robust or malnourished relationship I have with the creative process. For the first time, at twenty, I attempted to articulate my understanding of transpersonal psychology and my relationship to spirit and psyche. I will share selected excerpts of the paper with you here (Tuschman 2004).

> The unconscious has the tendency to speak to us in imagery and symbols as in dreams, and so the human urge to make art seems absolutely logical. It is, in many cases, an expression of the human desire to engage with his or her individual, as well as collective, unconscious. Thus, I may go even far as to say that artmaking is an attempt to extend our dream life into waking life, allowing our conscious mind to engage with the unconscious mind through a shared language of symbols and imagery.
>
> I should clarify before going further that when I refer to artmaking, I refer to the spontaneous process of mark-making, whether it is in drawing, painting, sculptural form, or simply scratching lines into a surface, in which the discovery is more important than actualizing a pre-prescribed representation, and risk-taking is more important than adhering to an accurate technique. It is only through this venturing into the unknown that one will come upon something authentic, a truthful message from the unconscious.

Willow: What you're writing feels very connected to how I just characterized the entirety of my work over the last three years, when I had to describe it in my contract renewal application. And I find as I'm teaching these two classes—"The Unconscious as Personal and Social Process" on the one hand and "The Transpersonal" on the other—that I've been engaged in that dialectic, between what we regard as the unconscious and what we regard as the transpersonal, for the last couple of years. I feel like the indivisibility of the unconscious and the transpersonal, which can be expressed as "the nondual un/conscious," is really the co-emergence of what is in shadow (the unconscious) and what is illuminated (consciousness). What you just wrote, what you just voiced, is like an ambassador of that indivisible reality. And this is just one languaging of it as the "nondual un/conscious," and I would love to write about that in our book.

Eva: It's interesting to read something I wrote when I was crossing the threshold from adolescence into young adulthood. I appreciate the young woman who was exploring these ideas and attempting to articulate connections for the first time.

Willow: Very beautifully, too.

Eva: Thank you. I'll continue reading from a different section:

> Like Jung, the act of artmaking, from furious scribbling with charcoal to the piecing together of a collage, has offered me a process of "finding imagery" amid ambiguous emotions. It has offered me a means of play and experimentation outside the structure of everyday life, and as a tool to recenter when I feel lost to myself. In short, making art, especially the act of making marks on paper, is the most direct way I engage my unconscious in waking life. It is the one realm in which I can safely welcome in the unknown.
>
> When I work with this open approach to creation I do not like to know what I am trying to do by visualizing a finished product. In fact, this not knowing is what thrills me and spurs me to keep going. It is what reminds me that I am part of a mystery, and this openness to the unknown evokes in me a sense of wonder and excitement. During this process, I am both creating the mystery, but the mystery is very much creating me. The invigorating play that transpires allows me to be able to be in this world, but also in another. I'm listening and responding to this other realm, learning to craft its energy.

Willow: Can you say those two lines again about the mystery in you and being crafted by the mystery?

Eva: "It is what reminds me that I am part of a mystery, and this openness to the unknown evokes in me a sense of wonder and excitement. During this process, I am both creating the mystery, but the mystery is very much creating me."

Willow: That's so beautiful.

Eva: Thank you. I'm going to skip ahead a bit now.

> When I'm immersed in the creative process, I'm not even aware that I'm engaging with something other. My conscious mind and my unconscious blend together. For the period that I'm playing and creating, I cease to remember that there ever was, or can be, a split in my psyche.

Willow: That's a lovely way to put it. You forget that there's ever a time that you weren't operating from the nondual un/conscious.

Eva: Yes. I think my twenty-year-old self had a strong experiential understanding of the nondual un/conscious.

> Balancing lines, dark and light, feeling texture, mapping out space, is such a deeply intuitive act for me. Through this activity, I'm able to enter completely into my true self. This is the self that has no I, the self

> that listens to something greater than the imminent anxieties of the day. My whole being, mind, and body, a clear conscious core is in service of something larger. This something is not characterized by a sensation of happiness or anger or sadness. Rather, it is completely valence-free. It just is. In this state of total equilibrium, I find center again.

I'm going to skip ahead by a few paragraphs.

> In this last year, I've identified a new theme in my dreams. I categorize these dreams as creativity dreams. I've experienced less than five of them, but each dream offers itself as a rare gift. The subject matter varies widely, though all of the dreams are linked by a powerful undercurrent of creative energy. Here is an example of a creativity dream I had in August 2004.

> *I'm filled with a sense of uncontainable excitement and drive to work. I'm sitting at a large wooden weaver's loom. I begin without hesitation to weave ecstatically. I throw the shuttle through the loom, flying it back and forth. I instinctively know the rhythm for the pattern I am making. "Under two, over three, under one, over two," I count aloud. My friend stands over my shoulder as I show him how to weave the pattern. The threads are exquisite, all varying shades of white. We decide to make a sculptural hanging with the gaps between the threads. The excitement of the weaving only increases, becoming at once fun and intensely life-affirming. Mostly, I am just so happy to know how to weave and to be working on this large project.*

At the time of this dream, I had no experience in my waking life of weaving. As a young woman, my mother was a weaver's apprentice in Denmark, so I have heard a lot about that time in her life.

Willow: Beautiful.

Eva: I'll continue on from there:

> I awoke from this dream feeling incredibly empowered, for it had connected me to a life force dwelling within that does not often get to express itself in waking life. What is perhaps most fascinating about this dream is that I'm not a weaver. I have never weaved before or even sat at a weaver's loom. But through this symbolic language of dreams, I experienced the archetypal energy of the weaver. Embodying this timeless energy, I was able to connect to a part of myself that is an instinctual creator.

Willow: I am appreciating how the luminous nondual un/conscious, which I describe as the interpenetrating continuum of unconscious consciousness ←→ conscious unconsciousness[1] (as a Bionian double arrow—which signifies that the element on one side of the arrow is indivisible from the element on the other side of the arrow, and that each element variously constitutes and becomes the other in its dynamic nature), can communicate an experience that is so utterly transcendent of the experience of the self, and that in the dream presence, the luminosity that transcends personal egoic experience can come through.

Eva: Absolutely, that's beautifully described. I'll skip ahead.

> I believe that working with the creative process over the course of a lifetime offers just as much a spiritual path toward individuation as a religion or psychoanalysis might provide. I should preface this by saying that one should never take their art too seriously, however, by deeming it overly precious, which I think can easily happen when one superimposes the one-sidedness of their ego onto the entirety of their work.
>
> I'm more concerned with the creative process, void of a teleological goal, with all its fluidity, mistakes, discoveries, destruction, fruition, and continual transformation. More than anything, the creative process is a practice of awakening, listening, being present and learning to appreciate the coexistence and perpetual shifts and opposites. In short, choosing to create is choosing to be alive to yourself as an individual.

I'll move ahead to the next dream. I'm skipping a few pages. "Fall quarter of this year, I had a powerful dream that speaks of this tension …" I believe I was describing the tension of studying art history and the critique of art, as opposed to the experience of making art, and the remove of that; being only in academic relationship to artmaking was very frustrating for me.

> *In the dream, I found myself in a foreign part of campus looking down from a high ledge at a large stone castle-like building. The castle was surrounded by beautiful gardens, and though its facade was old, inside the building, it was renovated and quite modern. Through the windows, I could see a printing press, large white studio spaces, and people pulling prints. I asked the woman who was with me, an administrator from the university, what was down there, and if I could go and look inside and participate. She promptly said no and explained that this was a private institute, costing several thousand dollars more in tuition.*

I'll pause there. I go on to explore what my "inner administrator" was communicating, the impediments she was constructing. Over the course of the last two decades, hidden art studios continue to show up in my dreams. Sometimes I can tour the spaces, feeling into a sense of wonder, excitement, and inspiration. I am on the verge of participation or readily engaging in creative process. Other times, I discover a hidden studio only to learn that it is off limits and I can't access the entrance.

Willow: It's so interesting. So one dream is where you're engaged in creative process, and the other is where you are wanting to gain access to the creative process, but somehow barred from it.

Eva: Yes, there is enthusiasm compounded by trepidation, restriction. "Will I be an imposter in this space? Will I be allowed entrance? Do I belong there?" I recall that I had applied to art school after my freshman year at Stanford, and I was accepted and then turned them down to return to Stanford. My own "inner administrator" shut off access to the full expression of my artist self. Variations on these themes have continually reappeared in my dreams over the last two decades. It's as though Psyche knows when I am distant from my creative life. Psyche shows me a hidden studio where other artists are actively making things, reminding me: "This is still available to you. You just have to figure out how to enter into it." Dreams illuminate a helpful tension. Something intrapsychically is off balance. The tension invites me to reunite with soul's calling.

Willow: How would you speak to the dreamer who is wondering how to enter into it? What would you advise her?

Eva: The first thing that comes to mind is to acknowledge that Psyche is already creating these beautiful and evocative dreams. So active and alive, Psyche conjures these dream experiences for me to viscerally remember the creative spirit existing within. This is the mystery—and the grace—of dreaming: Psyche offers an experience, a mirror, an emotional truth, as if by magic. The dream presents an invitation, reminding me to return to a part of me that is always accessible, no matter how long it has been dormant. Even when I ignore my creative life, it's still waiting for me to rekindle my relationship with it. And that's what gives me spiritual energy. That's what enlivens my soul. When I malnourish it, my soul suffers. Typically, that's when I notice myself feeling more depressed, perhaps more anxious, numb, or disconnected from life.

Willow: So plugging into creativity is plugging into psyche, soul, spirit.

Eva: Absolutely. I can look back at different periods of my life where my relationship to creativity has thinned and fragmented for different reasons. When I wrote this paper at age twenty, I was privileging rationality because of academic rigors, the ethos of an institution. Certainly this kind of learning has its place, yet I longed to also be in touch with my creative instinct. To ignore it was super detrimental.

Willow: I hear the importance of listening to the dreams that are beckoning you to access creativity, to not be locked out but opening to psyche, soul, spirit in order to listen to that deeply intuitive self—that deeply intuitive soul.

Eva: Yes. And as I reflect, there has been an evolution of the dream: Not only do I discover the secret art studio from the exterior, but I'm also able to enter into the interior and explore and move around the space and feel a sense of awe and excitement. I'm not locked out, and it's always kind of a surprise, like, "Oh, I didn't know this was here! Can I give myself permission to participate?"

Willow: So closing question. How would you, in this moment, give Psyche permission to participate? What would you say to her?

Eva: That's a beautiful question. I would tell her: You don't need permission, because it is your birthright. You came here to allow the creative spirit to move through you, to be in relationship and dialogue with it. And if and when I shut that valve off, that's a recipe for feeling numb and disconnected from life. I always have access to the creative spirit. The question is: Will I pay attention and make it important? Because it's a vital nutrient of what makes me want to stay awake to this experience of being alive.

Willow: Thank you.

Reflections Half a Lifetime Later

In many ways, the seeds for the book you now hold in your hand—and my path toward becoming a depth psychotherapist—were planted through the writing of this term paper more than twenty years ago. Intellectually and spiritually, I grappled with the material: I cared deeply about the ideas, so much so that I asked for an extension on the paper so that I could continue to articulate reflections and connections as authentically as possible. Academia, imposing rubrics of assessment, employed perfectionism, often hijacking and scrutinizing the process. I admire the young woman who wanted to give voice to nonlinguistic dimensions of her experience: the flow states that danced between her unconscious and conscious, as she followed her intuition, allowing mystery to inform her explorations.

I believe my younger self was intimately in touch with intuitive forms of knowing or what we might refer to now as feminine wisdom. She naturally understood how to be receptively open to the imaginal field. If anything, she was perhaps too porous to the unconscious as her dreamlife overflowed and sometimes overwhelmed her. But she also participated actively in a call and response, collaboratively listening to the unconscious and responding in turn through animate mark-making and discoveries of latent images.

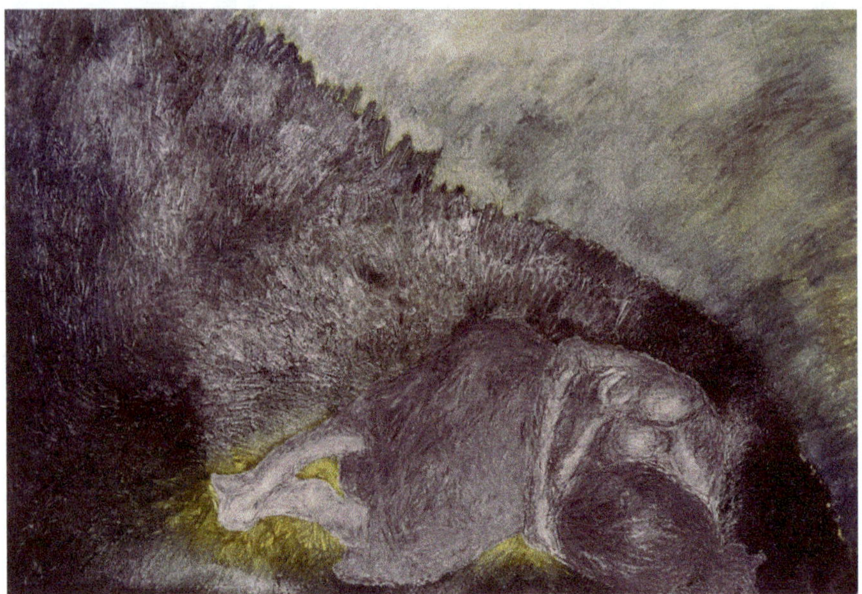

FIGURE 4.1 Oil stick and graphite on paper (1999)

When I was fifteen years old, I created this large drawing (Figure 4.1), an image of myself being overtaken by a tidal wave. This arose from a recurring dream of the same nature: *Helpless against the powerful forces of the ocean, I was repeatedly engulfed by a giant wave.* As an adolescent, I was relatively new to the depths of the unconscious. I had not yet cultivated wise ways of communicating with the unconscious's dynamic energy. Instead, I was "lost at sea," easily submerged, prone to drowning. Yet, in the process of creating this image of the dream, my power returned to me—I believe it was Jung's notion that we can "live the dream onward" by learning to actively collaborate with the unconscious in waking life. Dreams have awakened me, sometimes ferociously, sometimes exquisitely, to psychic undercurrents I've yet to fully acknowledge and integrate. Through the process of making marks, I transfer images from the dream realm into greater waking consciousness. This practice is not only enlivening, but also illuminating. The dream material, vivified, evolves; archetypal energies dance and transform. I discover new meanings, directions, and possibilities.

Artmaking, for me, provides the sacred meeting place between the unconscious and conscious, or as Willow expressed, "the nondual un/conscious." On these grounds, my psyche dances effortlessly between realms. Sometimes, dreams directly inspire the images that emerge; other times, soul guides me into the unknown and the image surfaces mysteriously. The latter was true for the following image (Figure 4.2), created when I was eighteen years old, the summer before entering college. Primitively stitched together are two parts, concealing a luminous core.

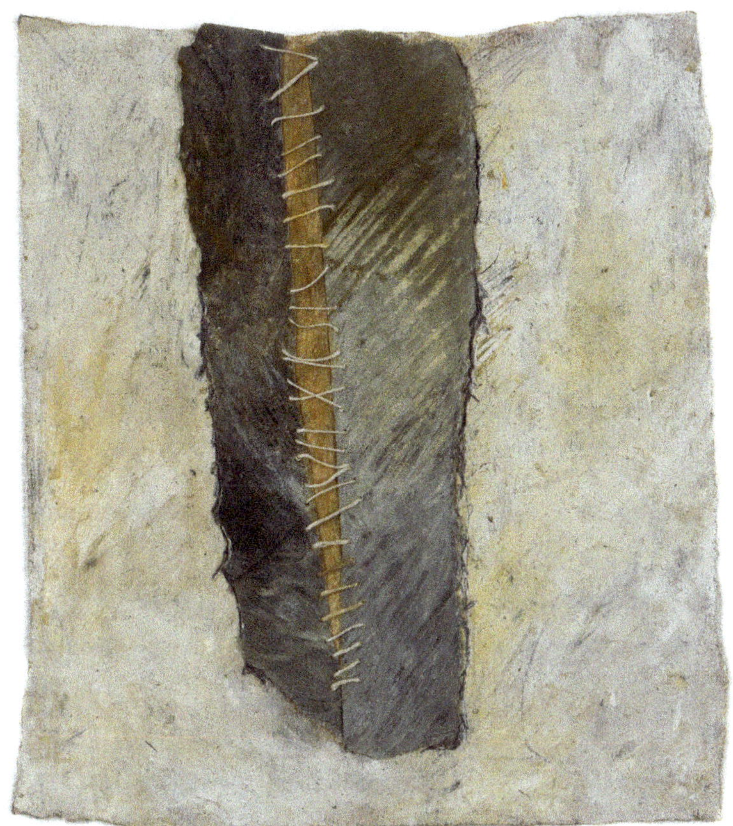

FIGURE 4.2 *Soul Sutures.* Oil stick, graphite, and thread on paper (2002)

Although seemingly simple, this image feels central to my soul's quest in this lifetime. It emerged intuitively before I could know its potential meanings. In some ways, it speaks of the union of opposites and the integration of the whole. In her book, *The Dreaming Way*, Toko-pa Turner writes: "Through a delicate alchemy of focus and receptiveness, Wisdom delivers us from the roiling of opposites into paradox. She gives us the ability to embrace *bothness,* releasing the need for a duel between contraries, so we can rest in their symmetry. From this relational ground comes a surge of energy" (2024, p. 61).

When I recently shared this image with my own psychotherapist, he entitled the piece *Soul Sutures*. This felt so right. The soul seeks the suturing of opposites; wisdom helps us to embrace *bothness,* as Turner writes. My younger self was beginning her journey to integrate seemingly opposing parts of her identity into a coherent self. And still, this quest for integration continues in midlife.

By yoking my body with my heart and my imagination, artmaking has been my soul's most fluent language. Whether through dance or song, poetry or sculpting, creative practice becomes a conduit for spirit as we navigate our earthbound lives. In a March 2025, seminar entitled *Arts and Practices: Creativity and Resilience in Times of Chaos and Crisis*, the storyteller and mythologist Michael Meade (2025) stated that "a practice is a way of continually resurrecting the essence of oneself." Practices, Meade asserts, are "ancient as a source, immediate as an expression … [allowing us to] blend our earthiness with our heavenly longings."

Dreaming by itself is not a practice. Psyche generously and mysteriously graces us with the gift of images each night. As Willow has articulated in our conversations, Psyche prolifically manifests "original artistry." Choosing to receive and unpack these gifts, even the ones that come in the form of nightmares, can become a spiritual practice. I believe strongly that when dreams illuminate tension, they are helping to bring us back in touch with soul, our wiser self. We can learn to open our heart-mind-spirit to the mercurial, luminous, awe-inducing, quizzical, sometimes terrifying tableaus that Psyche curates for us. Practicing reverence, we can receive and honor Psyche's original artistry. We can actively collaborate through our own artistic practices, through the writing of a poem or a song verse, an expressive movement, a sculpted object, an altar, or a painting. If we engage the creativity naturally pouring through our dreams, our lives become enriched with Psyche's wisdom, and in turn, our creative practices can feed and inform our dreams in an ever-expanding symbiotic relationship. No longer is there a distinct split between our unconscious and conscious. Creative practice invites us to play, to explore, to exist freely in the nondual un/conscious.

At this stage in my life, I no longer view my dreams as "other" or distinct from my lived waking experience; I include and embrace them as part of my phenomenological reality. For example, at age twenty, because I sat at a loom and ecstatically weaved in a dream, that archetypal energy now exists within me. In dreams I have carried a child in my womb, given birth, nursed a baby; I have died and been resurrected countless times; I have swum in the depths of the ocean with whales, shape-shifted into birds and wild cats. These experiences, transcending my small self or ego, live fully and fluidly in my cells and being.

When we welcome our dream life into our waking life we venture into the unknown. Art practice, an expression of spirit, a bridge between worlds, initiates deeper intimacy with soul. We need not necessarily interpret our dreams, but simply be open to the dynamic energies and possibilities that flow through them. Currently, my art practice involves forming wet earth into vessels (Figure 4.3). Just as I am shaping the clay, the process is very much shaping me. Through the craft of vesseling, I form organic spaces that can hold all that is still unripened. Fire and heat initiate the malleable earth into vessels that are at once strong and fragile, ancient in practice and alive in expression, containing alchemy within.

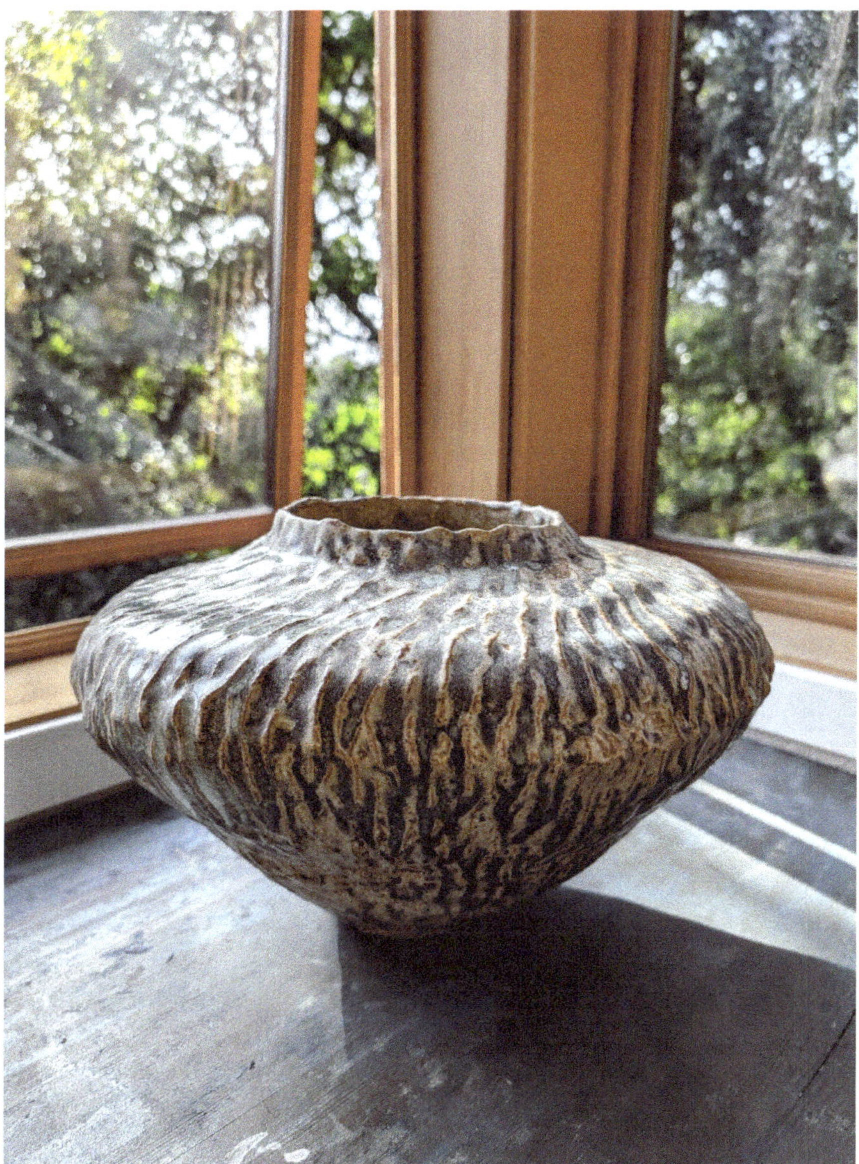

FIGURE 4.3 *Handbuilt Vessel* (2025)

The ceramicist M. C. Richards (1989), in her seminal book, *Centering*, which explores the poetry and metaphor of centering clay on the wheel, wrote about the importance of "not knowing and trusting simultaneously." So it is with dream practice. We enter the mystery, listen closely, and trust Psyche's wisdom to transform us.

Post-Script Dialogue

Willow: One of the amazing things about this writing is the way that you hold your younger self with such respect and care and allow yourself to honor not only her exactly in her nascent developmental space, but also the complete perfection of her as she is in you now and as she was then. I'm wondering if you can say something about honoring the timelessness of the soul in honoring this piece of writing.

Eva: I so appreciate you bringing the timelessness of the soul into the conversation. When I was nineteen, I took a leave of absence from Stanford and matriculated in an art program on a small island in Greece. It was a risk toward self-authorship, a distinct departure from socially defined expectations. Living abroad on my own was a very seminal experience for me: Through daily discipline, I wrote and worked on my art, developing both an intimacy with my inner life and a fidelity toward creative practices. I recall a very distinct memory that arose during this sojourn abroad: I felt like my soul was as ancient as it would ever be. It didn't matter that I was not yet even twenty; my relationship to soul felt timeless.

When I returned to Stanford and wrote this paper, the ideas that I attempted to articulate are ones that I deeply respect now. I honor, and even revere, my younger self who was grappling with those ideas and feelings, wanting to bring them forth. There is no hierarchy, meaning I do not diminish the expressions of my twenty-year-old self. She was channeling soul's wisdom, which was deep and transpersonal and eternal. This wisdom is just as relevant to me now at age forty-one and will be just as relevant to me in my last days of existence.

Willow: Part of what I appreciate about the path of this book is how we are learning from the timelessness of the soul as psyche is expressed through all these different nested dreamtimes of different ages and creative works. And how we can think of different ages themselves as different waking dreams. The waking dream of twenty, in this case that you're revisiting.

Eva: I know it can be a cliché when people say, "You're such an old soul." But I do think that there's something to be said for the soul being as old as it ever will be from the beginning.

Note

1 Psychoanalyst Christopher Bollas (1987) captures a meaningful dimension of this interpenetration of the un/conscious with his term "the unthought known."

References

Bollas, C. (1987). *The shadow of the object: Psychoanalysis of the unthought known*. Columbia University Press.

Meade, M. (2025, March). *Arts and practices: Creativity and resilience in times of chaos and crisis* [Seminar]. https://www.mosaicvoices.org/

Richards, M. C. (1989). *Centering in pottery, poetry, and the person*. Wesleyan University Press.

Turner, T. (2024). *The dreaming way: Courting the wisdom of dreams*. Her Own Room Press.

Tuschman, E. (2004). *Hearing imagery, feeling the invisible: An exploration of inner knowledge, archetypal energy and the relationship of the creative process with the unconscious* [Unpublished manuscript]. Stanford University.

5

OTHERS

Learning from Multiple Selves

In this chapter, Willow explores the mystery that we are to ourselves through a nighttime dream that points to multiple dimensions of self in both hidden and lucid conversation with one another. The nighttime dream, four days before her fifty-third birthday, figures an ego ideal, a persecutor, and a breakdown. At first, the voice of the soul is not heard. Then, through dream dialogue and further dream reflection, the transcendent and emergent self comes into being, by recognizing, centering, and listening to the voice of the soul harbored and encrypted by the dream. What was "Other," now apprenticed, becomes merely unfamiliar and, through practice, ultimately relatable. We contemplate the importance of beginner's mind in clinical work, and in the process, introduce a method of the grace of dreaming—namely, the caesura of the *dream navel* and the *dream umbilicus*, two ideas introduced by Sigmund Freud in his 1899 *Interpretation of Dreams*.

A Nighttime Dream: Jennifer One-as-silk

Four days before my fifty-third birthday, I had the following dream …

> *"Jennifer One-as-silk"—"amazing therapist and professor of an amazing PsyD program at Naropa University"—is leaving her position. She has a twin, who also runs the clinic of students-in-training.*
>
> *I have a breakdown consisting of the "confused gears" of the gold Toyota that I drive—a car that was gifted to me by my mother. I wander into Jennifer's suburban house in Marin, California, and join the students-in-training for support. Later I reveal that I am a longtime therapist and not a beginner.*

DOI: 10.4324/9781003591863-6

I tell Jennifer One-as-silk that I look forward to reading her writing. She looks at me with a penetrating gaze and expresses through her eyes alone that "it's all right here" in her present-moment embodied communication.

There is a woman, another therapist, in conflict with me. We try to process. I am livid. She outs me for my breakdown.

A Dream Dialogue

As context for the dream, I was a graduate student from 1996–1999 and then an adjunct professor from 2000–2007 at Naropa University—a Buddhist-inspired university in Boulder, Colorado. Although Naropa does not have a PsyD (Doctor of Psychology) program in "real life," I am currently a professor and director of clinical training in a PsyD program in clinical psychology at the California Institute of Integral Studies in San Francisco, California.

Willow: This dream occurred four days before my fifty-third birthday in 2023. So I had the dream on July 24, 2023.

This feels like a really rich dream with many facets of self. And what stands out for me in this moment is the expression from Jennifer One-as-silk where she says, through her eyes alone, "it's all right here." I'm struck—only in this moment in verbalizing it to you, Eva—that there's the double entendre of that statement. That it's all *right here*: that everything is here. And, at the same time and on another level, it's *all right* here. It's okay here.

It feels like both of these expressions are quite powerful and inextricably linked. On the one hand, the dreamer is really saying: "There's no need to go into the future. There's no need to produce anything, including writing. There's no need to look to some object of consciousness that's other than what's exactly here in this moment, beheld in the gaze of my eyes." And, in fact, the dreamer doesn't even need language of any kind. It's through her penetrating gaze that she expresses her present-moment embodied communication, the transmission of her revelation.

And so it feels to me like the dream carries this powerful recognition that it's all *right here—everything is present here in this moment*. And it's *all right* here—*it's okay here*.

This dream occurs in the presence of psychology teaching students *and* having a breakdown. It feels like Jennifer One-as-silk is also responding to that breakdown within her statement that it's *all right here*; *it's okay to be human*.

The dream is saying, It's okay to be broken. It's okay to be brokenhearted. It's okay to be broken down. It's okay to be the one who's not writing, the one who's not teaching, the one who's not practicing psychotherapy; it's okay to be the one who is just *here*. Just dwelling here; just existing here, exactly as you are. It's *all right here*. There is nothing missing within you. The dreamer is offering that recognition to the one who feels terrorized and terrified of being outed for her breakdown. Rather than being a persecutory figure—like the last therapist in the dream, the therapist Jennifer One-as-silk is in conflict with—instead what is offered in the dream is the message that *it's all right here*. It's okay to be human, to be broken, to have confused gears.

Eva: I feel like this dream is such an incredible gift, given to you by Psyche in preparation for your birthday. The timing as such feels quite salient to me. I always think that dreams leading up to one's birthday are hearkening back not only to the last year, but also to this whole developmental evolution of who you have become through Psyche taking inventory in this moment of time. The dream is asking the question, "Who am I becoming?" And what I love about Psyche's cleverness is that she's providing you with all of these different parts within yourself as they're trying to figure out which one is leading the way forward. And I think of the car in the dream, as this literal vehicle of movement into the future. It's the vehicle as self and as your coalition of parts. And right now, that vehicle is feeling confused. It's stuck.

Willow: The gears were literally stuck.

Eva: Yes.

Willow: That sticking of the gears landed me in front of Jennifer One-as-silk's suburban house.

Eva: Yes. For readers who may not know, the suburban house in Marin County, California, as a dream symbol, has the significance of attaining a certain level of success in the world, at least on the material level—a sense of having "made it" in terms of the San Francisco Bay Area lifestyle. And this symbolism certainly matches one aspect of the symbolism of her name, right? Jennifer *One-as-silk*. It's like perfection.

There's not a wrinkle in sight. She is "one as silk."

Willow: I was just going to comment on that, that Jennifer One-as-silk embodies an ego ideal of mine—my conscious ego ideal, which is not actually wholeness.

Eva: Absolutely.

Willow: And, to add further complexity, I can say that Jennifer, one of my middle names, was the name I went by in my youth. I didn't start going by my first name, Willow, until I was twenty-two.

The dream seems to represent, as you rightly said, a kind of wholeness because it includes all facets of the self.

Eva: Yes. And as I experience it in the dream, these different facets of self are vying for space and recognition. The therapist who wants to out you for the breakdown—that definitely feels like a shadow part that is going to expose something within you that may not look professional. It may not look coherent. Certainly not "one as silk." It's messy.

Willow: Fragmented.

Eva: Yes. But before I go on, I'm just curious, as you revisit the dream today, what resonates feeling-wise most for you?

Willow: What most resonates is just those two parts. When I had the dream, I was actually primarily reverberating with the ego ideal as a kind of super ego, a kind of pretense. And at the same time, I was also resonating with that ego ideal as its own kind of persecutory figure—persecutory because she's something, or someone, I can't live up to. Whereas the therapist whom I was in conflict with in the dream was another kind of persecutory figure in the sense of exposing or shaming me. And I think when I woke up from the dream, those were the two parts that I felt the residue of, that I was most aware of.

And now, two months later, almost to the day, what I'm really struck by—perhaps because of time and space, and also in no small part because of being in your receptive presence with the dream and knowing I've been able to bring the dream here to our dream dialogue, what stands out is that it's all *right here*. Everything is here. There's no place you need to go. There's no other place. And it's *all right* here. It is okay here. It's okay to be on this earth, in this body, in this mind, in this psyche, in this dance of life, in this expression of humanity on the planet.

Even with all that is broken and tortured and fragmented and suffering, all of that is acknowledged in the broken-downness, in the confused gears. That isn't denied or diminished or minimized. But nevertheless, there's a kind of wholeness of saying, it's all right here.

Eva: I feel like I'm experiencing the transmission through you, through Jennifer One-as-silk. A transmission that I actually really needed to hear today, after the challenging week that I've been through. That the broken parts, the confused parts, the grieving, messy, guilty parts … that it's all okay. So I'm appreciating the wisdom of the dream reverberating outward and toward me, which feels like a double gift.

In one sense, it is your dream. Psyche couldn't have created this dream specifically for anyone else. And yet the dream wisdom is wisdom that I need to hear as well.

Willow: That's beautiful. I appreciate in this moment how the transmission, as you say, of the dream from our psychotherapeutic lens, recognizes how you're like a mirror to me in the realization of the dream. But from the spiritual sense, as a spiritual container, the dream is an offering to us both.

Eva: Absolutely.

Willow: And I appreciate both of those lenses of the dream—individual and collective. How we are mirrors to one another from that psychotherapeutic space, how the dream is quite individual, and from the spiritual space, on a collective level, how the dream is just an offering from Psyche to psyches.

Eva: Beautifully said. And as you read the dream again today, for the second time in our dream conversation, I was definitely feeling, within myself, those parts that are struggling for space or recognition, the parts that don't want to be exposed or outed, and the amount of energy it takes to keep them orderly or have them quiet down. It's very striking to me.

The one who appears to be the super-ego ideal is actually the one who is most embodied, ultimately, who says: there's nothing beyond yourself that you need to figure out; you don't need to keep becoming or striving or accomplishing.

I'm not sure what to make of that, but it just really strikes me that she could have been a really scary figure, demanding a lot of perfection in your presentation. And yet she surprises us in the dream by actually being almost like this Zen master or spiritual teacher who illuminates enlightenment in *this moment*. It's nothing beyond you. It's right here, right now.

Willow: And the dreamer is not caught in the intellect's enterprise of language, of immanent or transcendent, here or there. Rather, the dreamer embraces that it's just literally all *right here*. And she doesn't get caught in the eye of the dream, doesn't get caught in the eddies of intellectual thought. The dreamer doesn't get caught in diversions or puzzles. Truth is very clear between the dreamer and the dream figures.

From this standpoint, in receiving the dream, there isn't a need for defense. I think that's one thing I'm struck by in the dream and in our sharing of it in this moment. The dream figure that I also was, the "other therapist" who was in conflict with me—to me, that very figure is an expression of the dream around defense. And as we hold it together now, as we receive the dream in this moment, in the afterwardness of the dream, the exchange between the one who has experienced breakdown and Jennifer One-as-silk is an undefended clear exchange.

Eva: One-as-silk is just this pure sense of unity.

Willow: I really appreciate the double entendre that you're pointing out in her name. That on the one hand there's the sense of the inhuman persecutory perfection of "no wrinkles, no flaws." And, on the other hand, as you're pointing out, there's the silk of the caterpillar-into-butterfly—the vessel of the cocoon in which one is born and transfigured. And that silk of the cocoon is—conveyed as you invoke the language of pure and genuine—not actually artifice.

Eva: I think my understanding has also evolved through your telling of the dream today, as opposed to my previous reading of the dream. Several weeks ago after I read the dream for the first time, I thought, how does the one who is dreaming move forward in her life given these various dynamic parts within her? But in some sense, there isn't really a need to jostle for control of which part is going to lead anymore, as I'm hearing it, because—as you so beautifully shared—it's all "one-as-silk." It's all wrapped in this shroud of silk: all the confusion, the doubt, the defense. All aspects of self feel contained in this dream silk shroud.

Willow: I'm having a really meaningful association as you say the "silk shroud." I'm remembering a friend of mine, Bonnie Bostrom,[1] who's a painter and writer as you are and who is also a psychotherapist. Through our friendship, she attended a Women's Integral Life Practice seminar that I offered with two other teachers, many years ago, at Omega Institute in Reinbeck, New York. And Bonnie brought cotton shawls for each of us who were presenting. I still have my shawl. It was a beautiful offering of something that was both ornamental and comforting at the same time.

And the other association I'm having, in addition to that cotton shawl from Bonnie, is an association to an Indian blanket that was gifted to me when I ended my time as a psychotherapist at Puyallup Tribal Health Authority, at the Kwawachee Counseling Center in Tacoma, Washington, after I had been working there ten months. It was a traditional gift to give an Indian blanket as a blessing of arrival or departure. I cherish this beautiful blanket. And, again, it's something that is wrapped around a person as a kind of symbol, and there is also the actuality of being held in fabric, in protection, in a layer of protection and comfort and warmth and embrace. It's an embrace of clothing and cloth that is its own kind of material provision and spiritual transmission.

Eva: Beautiful. It's important to include these other associations and perspectives because if we were just looking at this dream through the lens of Western psychology, we could look at it, for example, through Internal Family Systems and see that each of these parts is vying for your control or attention. And that could be a useful rendering of the dream. That was my first reading of the dream—the sense of the professional self or the perfectionistic self or the judgmental self.

And yet, I'm also appreciating that we can find a place to settle into the dream, which I imagine for you as the dreamer is where the wisdom resides around feeling like there's an inclusion of all the parts—the wisdom that you can wrap all the parts up and be held in this one-as-silk shawl. And that way your professional self isn't having to repress the parts that feel messy.

It reminds me of a former supervisor of mine many years ago who said something to the extent that as therapists, it's not that we don't have our own challenges and personal problems in our lives, that we don't go through relational difficulties and losses and struggle with our own complexes. That's a given. But he said something to the extent that it's how we learn to relate to all of the different parts within us and that we're actively engaging our awareness that makes the difference. And I found that to be such a relief.

To use the language of your dream, it's not that we have to become a one-as-silk version of ourselves and live in a suburban house in Marin—although that sounds nice!—but there's still room for the parts that are rusty or out of gear or literally having the breakdown.

Willow: Yes. As you invoked Robin Bagai's quote that "Dreams…look backward and forward [at once] … they are sources of potential new births" (Robin Bagai, personal communication, seminar on Michael Eigen, November 1, 2020), I'm also reminded that I had a conversation with Robin recently where we were asking each other "What's your next writing project?" And he responded to me saying, "I don't know that I'll ever do another writing project again, and there's something very liberating in that." And I remember being shocked by his answer, because he's such an amazing, illuminating, beautiful writer and thinker and dreamer. And yet there was indeed something liberating in his transmission of that expression to me. And I feel like this realization is carrying through in the advent of this book project, *The Emotional Truth of Dreams*, in that there's something transforming for me about recognizing that it's not an imperative to write this book. It's a wish and desire. That desire to write this book is not principally coming from the place of trying to expand my professional self. That the desire to write this book is principally coming from a place of wanting to learn from the dreamer. The dreamer in me, the dreamer in you, the dreamer in us, and the dreamer who wants to be invited into this world through others as well.

Eva: And I would add, in addition to wish and desire, the call to listen to soul's expression. This isn't something that involves doing a bunch of research to advance or elevate your professional life for other people's approval. And that's so interesting because I'm actually now hearing echoes between the dream, which happened obviously before we decided to have this book be an expression of soul. And in a way, I feel like you're really listening to Jennifer One-as-silk's transmission in your decision to write the book as a call of the soul.

Willow: I was afraid to include Jennifer One-as-silk. I was afraid to include this dream in the former version of the book. I couldn't find a place for the dream. And now that it's no longer a book about a particular form of psychotherapy, but actually a book about learning from our dreams and learning from our soul—the mystery of the soul through the practice of listening to our dreams and writing them and speaking them and hearing our associations to them and questions about them—there's a place for this dream.

Eva: I would say a central place. In a way, it really does feel like this decision to include the dream here is a decision to really listen to soul and to trust in soul's expression, as opposed to following something you think you *should* be doing, something that the professional self should be achieving. Which isn't to say that the creation of this book won't also have professional value. I think it absolutely will.

It's just that we're not necessarily trained in terms of soul work in graduate school. Certainly that word, *soul*, didn't come up when I was a student at the Wright Institute, but I think that soul is what principally guided us to become clinicians. Yet soul wasn't ever spoken of at school. Somehow it was sort of taboo.

I'm curious about why that is—because the soul is always speaking to us and wanting expression. But often, I know for me, especially to get through a lot of my education, I had to turn the volume down on soul or intentionally reset my focus on being very theoretical. And being theoretical also has its place, but I do feel like there was something lost in the guiding spirit of it all.

And I certainly felt a tremendous loss of relationship to soul language as a student at Stanford University. That time in my life, I was experiencing a lot of depression and anxiety, which was certainly symptomatic of not really feeling like there was a place for soul and not a place for what Jennifer One-as-silk is saying. There was not a sense of it's all right here. There was not a sense that you have everything you need already. The difference between simply being and the drive to always be becoming something is a split I lived in college. So one of the things I take away from this dream is that there doesn't have to be all of this strife and struggle with all of our different internal parts.

Actually, it's all okay for them to coexist, and nothing's wrong with them having their own words and needs. I'm able to internalize the wisdom of the dream: all the parts within you can coexist.

Willow: I'm so glad that we returned to this dream today. If the book project had gone in its original direction, or if I hadn't been willing to have some level of reveal in sharing the dream, then we wouldn't be having this conversation and I would have just put the dream away. And I'm so grateful that there's this space between us and that it has allowed this dream to be shared, allowed for the ongoing emergence and evolution of the dream, if you will, in our own experience.

Eva: Thank you, Willow, for having the courage to let the dream fully live in open air and open space rather than tucking it into a notebook and coming back to it decades from now. Because I think the dream is only as potent and alive as one chooses to give it credence and values it with reverence. I think it's so easy to shy away from the power of a dream and not take it into full view because it can feel like, am I willing to really listen to the power of the dream? And more than that, am I willing to live from the power of the dream?

Willow: Beautiful. Thank you. Thank you so much.

Eva: Yes, thank you.

Dream Messages: Further Learning from the Mystery of the Soul

I have been terrified to share this dream. And, equally if not more so, I have been compelled to share this dream. And perhaps between the emotional truths of that terror and that desire, lies the grace of dreaming Jennifer One-as-silk.

Upon waking, I first imagined Jennifer One-as-silk as whom I wished to be. Yet I imagined her as Other, as someone to live up to. Yet, I am discovering, in listening and opening further to her, both in dream dialogue with Eva and in my reflections following that dialogue, that Jennifer One-as-silk is, in fact, a multifaceted and dynamic dream figure.

She is not a simple ego ideal, as I first imagined upon waking and holding and writing down the dream. She is not merely the self I would wish to be seen as. Rather, she can be read *simultaneously* as an idealized version of myself whom I would wish to be seen as, as a persecutory figure I cannot live up to, as a spiritual teacher who embraces both her ego and her transcendent self at once, and as a transcendent dreamer who is both a nascent, cocooned caterpillar and an emergent, burgeoning butterfly.

And the grace of dreaming is that I do not have to elevate one dimension or one version of the dreamer over another. The grace of this particular dream is that all facets of the dreamer—even the therapist I am in conflict with who would shame and humiliate me—have a place in dreaming as an expression of the spiritual psyche. I do not have to "integrate" all of these parts. I can allow all of these parts to dwell within me, as me, as multiplicitous as these parts are.

Although psychic organization certainly has its vital place in the process of psychotherapy, and psychic integration can be a meaningful part of that process, this dream is about something more foundational. It is about psychic recognition.[2] Before any organization or integration can take place, we have to know who lives here, in this house called Psyche. This dream is welcoming all of these disparate parts within me, when I hold the dream from the vantage of the embracing soul. The process of receiving the dream, writing it, sharing it, dialoguing about it, and reflecting further on it, allows for that soul embrace.

And this wisdom of the dream, this embrace, scares me. Really, I think, can I actually allow all of these parts to coexist within me? I do not have to banish the part that has experienced breakdown? I do not have to heal her? I do not have to complete her? I do not have to make her whole? She can be broken within me and still I can include her, embrace her, accept her? This is indeed what the soul is teaching me in this dream, supported through Eva's trusted and caring, natural therapeutic presence, which, in turn, supports my own.

I cannot live up to the ideal of Jennifer One-as-silk because she is not real. And because of this, when I get in touch with this fact, I can see that she actually persecutes me. In a sense, she doesn't allow me to exist as I am. She doesn't ever breakdown. She doesn't fragment, dissolve, deconstruct, change, become. She doesn't disappear. In this sense, the sense of ego ideal, she is a construct, not a living being.

The energy it takes to separate the ideal self from the whole self is exhausting. The whole self cannot exclude her any more than she can be reduced to her.

The soul's call in this dream is to *allow* the ideal self, even to *celebrate* her, while also recognizing her as ultimately illusory. But this dream discernment is not as simple as recognizing ego as illusory. The grace of this dream is that ego has a rightful place in the constellation of the self. Even as ego is not the whole self. And even as ego is neither a static nor a solid self.

Similarly, the wounded self, the self that experiences breakdown, is not simply suffering or confused.[3] She too has a rightful place in the constellation of the self. She contains her own questions and experiences and understandings and wonderments. The tale of breakdown, of trauma, is not the whole story of the self. Yet the wounded self harbors many illuminations for the transcendent self to learn from. As one example, the stuck gears of the Toyota are what places Jennifer One-as-silk in relationship to the breakdown as well as to the community of students at the clinic.

A message of the dream is that it is *all right* to be here—broken down before the Marin suburban house that is linked to the student clinic. And that in this dream place, it is *all right here*—there is no need to elevate one dimension of the dream above another, no need to place one dimension of the dream beneath another. Each has its rightful place in the spiritual psyche, in existence, in being and becoming. The movement of Jennifer One-as-silk from an Other within who is both cherished and feared, to a host of multiple selves that collectively experience pain, confusion, wisdom, transcendence, and acceptance, is part of the mystery and learning of the soul's dream.

Another theme, another contemplation, of the dream I wish to turn to is that of what in Buddhism is often referred to as "beginner's mind." In the dream, recall, *I have a breakdown consisting of the "confused gears" of the gold Toyota that I drive—a car that was gifted to me by my mother. I wander into Jennifer's suburban house in Marin, California, and join the students-in-training, for support. Later I reveal that I am a longtime therapist and not a beginner.*

Here, the wounded self who experiences breakdown wanders and then *joins the students-in-training for support*. Further, that very wounded self *later reveals that I am a longtime therapist and not a beginner.* In reflecting further on the dream, it seems that Psyche, who we can understand as ever and always the spiritual psyche (see Pearson & Marlo, 2021), brilliantly and creatively unites beginner's mind with longtime experience, holding them as nonseparate, even as the spheres of being a student-in-training and being a longtime practitioner are also distinguished in the dream.

As a professor of clinical and counseling psychology, I am aware that it has often been observed by senior clinicians and students-in-training alike that, from a systems perspective, in terms of how graduate students figure in relationship to community mental health clinics, the most inexperienced students are routinely assigned to work with the most profoundly disturbed and hard-to-reach clients. Understandably, this systemic practice of pairing clients most in need with students who lack clinical experience is often noted as a failing of the mental health system, both in the United States specifically and, more broadly, internationally as well. And certainly, from the perspective of education and practice, it would be ideal if those patients most in need were to receive care from the most experienced clinicians.

And yet, this dream is pointing to the wisdom of beginner's mind even as it also honors (and also casts suspicion on) longtime experience. In this respect, the dream points out that psychotherapy is ultimately and also foundationally conducted by a soul-to-soul connection (and disconnection) between the patient and the clinician that, in a meaningful way, prefigures education. And, in the dream, the longtime practitioner and professor in me is seeking refuge with the students-in-training. There is a refuge for me with the students-in-training who are working at the clinic. The implication of the dream is that the students-in-training implicitly allow for and receive the wounded self's breakdown, whereas the therapist who appears at the end of the dream "outs me for my breakdown"—unlike the students, she is shaming and not accepting. The implication in the dream is that the therapist's education and training have actually, ironically, dissociated her from breakdown. So, as I reflect further, it seems that the dream points me back to the essential healing ground of soul-to-soul exchange that is not dependent on training and education. And, in receiving this dream message, I am reminded that being a longtime therapist (at the time of this writing, I have practiced psychotherapy as a licensed clinician for twenty-five years) brings both the gifts of experience and the challenges of both witnessing and letting go of preconception, to invoke Wilfred Bion's work on having ideas in the mind that can preclude open awareness into the unknown.

Within this awareness of the healing resource of beginner's mind, I return to the dream's opening: *"Jennifer One-as-silk"—"amazing therapist and professor of an amazing PsyD program at Naropa University"—is leaving her position. She has a twin, who also runs the clinic of students-in-training.*

In this dream, I leave my position. I think "position" can be read as my role as a professor, my stance as a clinician, and my name. As I mentioned in the dream dialogue with Eva, *Jennifer*, one of my middle names, was the name I went by in my youth. I didn't start going by my first name, *Willow*, until I was twenty-two. Another realization this dream brings is that *Willow*, the name that I associate with my true self, with my authentic self, is the core therapist and healer in my work with patients. My professional name, *Doctor Pearson Trimbach*, is the name I associate with my professorial and clinical psychologist self. *Doctor Pearson Trimbach* is invaluable and essential in my roles of teaching and of doing psychotherapy, as an orienting, healthy, and supportive super ego. But in the dream, I am leaving this professional position of professor, in the sense of leaving orienting to this super ego as the core self. For it is *Willow* who experiences resonance with and empathy for patients on the felt level of life experience by connecting with my own. And, in parallel, my choice to let go of being called *Jennifer*, a middle name my parents chose for me, and my further choice in my twenties to go by my first name, *Willow*, represents a decision to jettison my parents' conception of me and to welcome my true self. All of these names are welcomed and challenged and also played with in the dream.

Yet, too, as the dream continues: *I have a breakdown consisting of the "confused gears" of the gold Toyota that I drive—a car that was gifted to me by my mother.* In this way, there is recognition in the dream that my mother offers me the gift of this vehicle, this multiplicitous self, this life. There is an embrace of the name that my mother gave me, *Jennifer*. And, further, the dream communicates that this gift of self, this gift of life, this *Jennifer One-as-silk* includes all aspects of the multiple self: the ego ideal, the persecutor, the breakdown/wounding/trauma, the transformative and emergent selves, and their embrace. There is no definitive meaning about my name in this dream, no ultimate interpretation, only endless emergent realizations that issue from it. I have many names, and my name changes depending on role and context, and the soul can both welcome, include, and also transcend all of these names. In this way, the dream welcomes me to just be *Willow*.

We all have multiple names. We all have multiple selves. And we all have parts of ourselves that we hold as Other within us. The grace of dreaming is that we can apprentice these others within and come to know them as dimensions of the soul.

In the Afterward of the Dream

After writing the dream messages, I go back to sleep. And in the dreamtime, I am visited by bizarre trickster dreams that, upon waking, leave me with the impression that the dreamtime is always generating more than we can imagine digesting, more than we can enter with consciousness. Upon waking, I feel visited by the truth that our dreaming is always more than we can fathom, that the imaginal realm is always greater than the known, and that we are ever bound to and beheld by the deeper layers of the mysteries of the soul.

The fact that we remain unknown to ourselves, in no small measure, is not cause for despair: that we are forever cast into the dreaming sea,[4] by day and by night, is cause for wonder.

Yet this being at sea is only part of dreaming. There too is a boat, a shoreline, and a safe harbor. Dream dialogue is like a boat. Dream messages are like a shoreline. Resting in these is safe harbor.

The practice of listening for the *Emotional Truth of Dreams* is *learning from the mystery of the soul*, which is a method of realizing the caesura of the dream navel *and* the dream umbilicus.[5] Simply put, I would offer that Sigmund Freud's (2010, p. 25) "dream navel"—which Freud defines as "a tangle of dream-thoughts which cannot be unraveled and which moreover adds nothing to our knowledge of the content of the dream"—intimates the hope and fear that the dream is, that we are, separate, temporal, and knowable. Whereas I would assert that Freud's (2010) "umbilicus of the dream"—the dream's connection to the unknown—touches the hope and fear that the dream is, that we are, continuous, infinite, and mysterious.[6]

Separating and joining these linked yet distinct realizations, this caesura invites the grace of dreaming. The mysteries of the soul can be realized even as they are yet unknown. We are both conscious and unconscious at once. To live this multiplicity, what I have previously called "enlightenment and endarkenment" (see Pearson & Marlo, 2021), what I refer to here as the *nondual un/conscious*, is to cultivate, simultaneously, reverence for the soul's profound intimacy *and* for the soul's eternal encryption.

Dreams encrypt the messages of the soul even as they unfold them. To learn from the mystery of the soul, by apprenticing our dreams, is like a game of hide and seek. Ultimately, the dream umbilicus remains hidden even as the dream navel is sought and found. Likened to the circular ouroboros—the timeless dragon snake who eats its own tail—learning from dreams is continuous even as their essential mystery is without end.

To open once again from embodied theory to essential practice, perhaps by illustrating the way in which our dream lenses (clear theoretical perspectives) can open new meaningful connections (associations and links), new revelations of the dream open into awareness. Namely, *One-as-silk* is the *khata*, a white (or multicolored) silk offering of respect and acknowledgment of being in the presence of the living Buddha/bodhisattva. This is a Buddhist ritual that Lama Palden Drolma taught us at Sukhasiddhi Foundation. Guided by Palden's teaching, I then presented a *khata* to Khenpo Tsültrim Gyamtso Rinpoche, when I first met Rinpoche and heard him teach the deity practice of *Chenrezig*, or *Avalokiteshvara*, Lord of Love (see Bokar Rinpoche, 1991, for meditation practice). This was in San Francisco, sometime around 2005 or 2006.

The khata symbolizes a recognition of purity, in the spiritual sense—the pure recognition of Oneness that is inseparable from the Many. Writing this just now, I am reminded of another approach of reverence that I made to another root teacher, Ken Wilber. After reading Ken's book *Grace and Grit,* as a new student at Naropa in 1996, about the life, love, and death of his beloved wife Treya Killam Wilber, I set this phrase from his writing to song and sent it to him with a note of gratitude: "Free the Many, Find the One, Taste the Many as the One." This too was a blessing. Who knows how this transmission of grace, between Ken and Treya, inspiring my song, now figures in the writing of this book? Khata and song, each offered from the genuine heart of recognition of a root teacher and the call of my soul to connect.

In this way, this dream of Jennifer One-as-silk is a dream of radical acceptance of the bodhisattva not as an Other within, but as One, who is Many, who is indigenous to the soul.

Notes

1 See https://www.bonniebostrom.com for Bonnie's luminous poetry, books, and paintings.

2 This emergent disposition in relationship to the dream is, upon consideration, a basis for what Michael Eigen has called, following Donald Winnicott, *psychic democracy*. See Fuchsman and Cohen (2021).

3 For a profound holding of the wounded self, see Kristeva (1997). For a further profound holding of the wounded self, see the forthcoming work, *The Luminous Wound*, by Therese Schroeder-Sheker. For access to this work, through music thanatology, see *Chalice of Repose Project* at https://chaliceofrepose.org/

4 See Willow Pearson and Eric Ramstad's *Dreaming Sea* [CD], from Unruffled Productions. You can retrieve it at https://www.lionessroars.org/music/dreamingsea, together with downloadable and streaming music services worldwide including Apple Music, SoundCloud, and Spotify.

5 See Daws (2009) for a theoretically elegant and beautifully clinically illustrated dream portal. Here, I read Daws expressing a kindred realization when he writes the following: "The dream can be viewed as a highly complex, infinitely structured and layered reality, reflecting a pre-Caesurian and Caesurian logic condensed into various endoscopic scenarios, unique to each person's psychological reality, constantly being transformed, and seeking ultimate reality or truth about the 'original situation'" (p. 30). And perhaps, we could link to what is offered here by also writing this as an "O-riginal situation," to denote Bion's "O." The original situation as conceived in this present work is not only the absent breast but also the caesura, both as a link between and shift from floating in a sonorous amniotic womb to self-emergence through a cut umbilicus and as one's Original Face, the face before both of your parents were born—in the sense of the Zen Buddhist koan pointing out one's unborn, undying Buddha nature arising and dissolving as one's unique self. The caesura of one's unborn, undying Original Face includes and embraces the absent breast and the cut umbilicus, free of reductionism or conflation. For a musical ode to Original Face, visit https://www.lionessroars.org/music/burning and scroll down to "Original Face."

6 To link Freud's writing of the dream navel and dream umbilicus with Grotstein's writing of the ineffable subject of being (the Dreamer who Understands the Dream or, more accurately, the Dreamer who Participates in the Dream), and the supraordinate subject of being (the Dreamer who Dreams the Dream) with Daws's pre-Caesurian and Caesurian dimensions of the dream, through my sense of this relationship between the dream navel and the dream umbilicus, and the realization of *nested dreams*, we could say: Dream

navel is linked with the ineffable subject of being (the Dreamer who Participates in the Dream and the Dreamer who understands the Dream), which is Caesurian logic; whereas Dream umbilicus is linked to the supraordinate subject of being (the Dreamer who Dreams the Dream), which is pre-Caesurian logic.

References

Daws, L. (2009). Dreaming the dream: In search of endoscopic ontology. *Issues in Psychoanalytic Psychology, 31*(1), 30.

Freud, S. (2010). *Interpretation of dreams: The complete and definitive text* (J. Strachey, Ed. & Trans.). Basic Books. (Original work published 1899.)

Fuchsman, K., & Cohen, K. S. (Eds.). (2021). *Healing, rebirth and the work of Michael Eigen: Collected essays on a pioneer in psychoanalysis*. Routledge.

Kristeva, J. (1997). Powers of horror: Approaching abjection. In K. Oliver (Ed.), *The portable Kristeva*, (2nd ed.). Columbia University Press.

Pearson, W., & Marlo, H. (Eds.). (2021). *The spiritual psyche: Mysticism, intersubjectivity, and psychoanalysis*. Routledge.

Rinpoche, B. (1991). *Chenrezig, lord of love: Principles and methods of deity meditation*. Clearpoint Press.

6

SURRENDER

Learning from Illness

This chapter explores the insights gleaned from a nighttime dream in which Eva loses a backpack symbolizing her core identities. The subsequent dialogue unpacks themes of loss, identity, and the potential for spiritual awakening when external supports are stripped away. Associations range from the intentional shedding of possessions to the forced displacement of refugees and the archetypal journey of the wanderer. The narrative then shifts to Eva's experience with unresolved illness, framed as a "beautiful nightmare." Drawing parallels between the surreal nature of dreams and the disorienting reality of living with a debilitating condition, she recounts her journey through medical gaslighting and the erosion of her former life. Embracing a "waking dream" perspective becomes a coping mechanism, fostering curiosity and detachment. The chapter further examines the liberating potential of dreams in extreme circumstances, citing the experiences of Auschwitz prisoners and Civil War soldiers who found solace and connection through shared dreamwork. Finally, the transformative power of a dream group in a women's maximum-security prison highlights how tending to dreams can foster self-awareness and agency even in confinement. The chapter concludes by emphasizing the boundless freedom offered by our dream lives, even when our waking realities are severely restricted.

Nighttime Dream

I am wandering through the holy city of Jerusalem. On my shoulders, I am carrying a very heavy backpack. I wonder why I am carrying so many heavy textbooks. I wander into a shop in the center of the ancient city. I place my backpack down to look at clothing. When I return to pick up the bag, it is gone. I look everywhere in the shop. I begin to feel panicked. I ask the shopkeeper if they have seen it. Then,

DOI: 10.4324/9781003591863-7

more agitated, I accuse them of taking it. I become distressed as I realize I have nothing: no wallet, no passport, no money, no identification, no phone, no books.

How will I ever find my way back home?

I head toward the cavernous hallway of the shop, determined to find my stolen bag. The shopkeeper declares that she never took the bag. She pulls out a rusty weapon, attacking me from behind, and we wrestle for control.

Dream Dialogue

Willow: What do you notice in your body as you access the dream in the present moment together?

Eva: Revisiting the dream, it truly feels like a lived experience in my body. I feel distressed at the sudden loss of everything that was holding my identity together in the bag.

Willow: Adding this new dimension of sharing our dreams through video rather than just voice, I'm able to resonate with the experience of physical tension as you relate the dream. I have my own personal associations to it. When I left Boulder and moved to Washington State, I let go of the vast majority of my personal belongings. It was the first time I had done that as an intentional shedding of material possessions. I am reminded of the freedom and terror in that process. A sense of release and unbinding of burden, of identity, and also simultaneously a clinging to it and questioning, "*Why did I do that*?"

Eva: There is a sense of security found in material belongings. They reflect our status. Especially as a wanderer, I feel safe if I carry these belongings on my back because I have some sense of knowing who I am wherever I go.

Willow: Another association I have to the dream is about the transmission of the Dharma from India to Tibet. I think of the yogi, Naropa, who let go of all of his Dharma texts as he was traveling and just carried what was inside of him. I can imagine how astonishing that must have been for a great scholar to release all of his precious books and to go forth only with what was in his heart, mind, and spirit.

Eva: I am reminded of the contemporary story of Yongey Mingyur Rinpoche, who slipped out of his monastery in the middle of the night, with the intention of spending the next four years on a wandering retreat, following the ancient practice of holy mendicants. He was a revered teacher, yet his goal was to discard his title in order to explore the deepest aspects of his being. When he no longer wore his robes, which signified his esteemed role, people didn't regard him with the same respect, which was extremely confronting for him. I also think about refugees who flee their homeland and are forced to leave behind their physical belongings. All they can transfer across borders is their ideas, values, and culture, which they carry invisibly within.

Willow: The themes of the refugee, the wanderer, the aescetic letting go of material possessions, all come to mind as archetypes within your dream.

Eva: Yes. It also seems that Psyche chose the geographic context very precisely for this dream.[1] Jerusalem is a holy city where seekers from all over the world go on pilgrimage. I myself went on pilgrimage there as a young woman in my twenties. Psyche situated the dream on holy ground.

Willow: … On holy ground letting go of your backpack … And then there's the conflict: the ruckus, the tussle between the shopkeeper and yourself, accusing the shopkeeper of stealing the backpack. I'm wondering what associations you have to that conflictual aspect of the dream.

Eva: I see the shopkeeper as illness personified, the way that she caught me off guard and attacked me from behind. There's a sense of being blindsided by it. We are wrestling for who has control of the situation. When illness suddenly hijacked my life in my mid-thirties, I was so distressed and shocked—my initial instinct was to fight it and reclaim control.

Willow: So as you continue to dream into the dream in this moment, with the shopkeeper figuring as illness,[2] what do you imagine would be the next movement of the dream?

Eva: What a beautiful question. I fearfully wonder in the dream: *How will I find my way home? How will I survive without the identities important to my ego? How do I navigate the unknown without my "book knowledge"?*

I'd like to imagine that I actually walk away entirely from the shop, that I don't engage in more self-defense, that I become a wanderer in the Holy Land. I reassure myself that I don't need to be frantically grasping for an old story of who I am. The material possessions are stolen and not coming back. Now I can come to know who I am in a deeper spiritual, immaterial dimension. The Holy Land is not such a bad place to find myself.

Willow: I'm wondering if there is an image or symbol of that home you are already in as you invite yourself to wander the Holy Land?

Eva: I can't think of a symbol per se; it's more a feeling of the shift from panic and distress to surrender and release. I think it was the Jungian psychologist Connie Zweig (2021) who, in her book, *The Inner Work of Age*, speaks about the transformation from "role to soul." *Role* being the identities and responsibilities I've held, and *soul* being the deeper dimensions of my being. The dream provides a mirror: *Who am I once my external identities are taken away? What is my relationship to soul without familiar roles?*

Willow: Do you have a sense of what medicine this dream offers to you in the present moment?

Eva: A beautiful question. I think the dream offers a window into what has been a harrowing six-year journey with complex unresolved illness up until now. The dream as medicine assists me in seeing clearly that this disorienting, wayward path, which has radically interrupted the trajectory of my life, has transformed me at a deep level. Being forced to surrender my career, my apartment, my independence as I fell ill was extremely confusing, as all initiations are. By necessity, I've had to search for a deeper understanding of who I am that is not represented in the accomplishments listed on my CV, nor can I find answers in the academic knowledge I've accumulated through my education and training. Living with a mysterious complex illness has been an entirely different sort of spiritual training that nothing in the backpack can easily solve. The dream provides a helpful mirror, illuminating what I've been living through in clearer terms.

The medicine of the dream is a gift because it helps me to witness my own process from a new vantage point. Yes, there have been unchosen changes in the physical realm of my life, but there has also been immense transformation in the spiritual, unseen realms as well. I thank Psyche for locating the dream in the Holy Land as I'm now more aware of the spiritual metamorphosis at a soul level.

Willow: Beautiful. Are there other thoughts, associations, reveries, links, connections about this dream that you want to include or speak to, touch on, or even questions that it opens?

Eva: I remember peering into the backpack and seeing these very big chunky academic textbooks that I don't think I've carried around since I was in college. These textbooks feel symbolic of the amount of discipline that I've engaged in my life to be studious and loyal to my studies. I thought that it was so clever of Psyche to tuck this symbol into the backpack because she's communicating, "This, too, isn't going to help you with what you're going through now."

I also smile that in the shuk (marketplace) I was looking for clothing, a symbol of how I represent myself outwardly to the world. Again, I'm reminded of the Rinpoche who gave up his robes: suddenly he's considered nobody, a beggar people ignore. I relate to this because when illness took away my career and other roles in my life, an existential question loomed: "What is my value to others when I can no longer work? How do I value myself when I surrender particular titles that once garnered respect?" And that can be really confronting in our ableist society that places so much emphasis on how you're contributing to the capitalist system. The backpack contains socially defined identities and suddenly I'm without its contents to rely on. I'm forced to contend with so much loss simultaneously; it's frightening. But also as you mention earlier, there can be an element of liberation once we learn the practice of surrender. My soul is neither defined by my outer appearance, nor by what I carry in my backpack. I deeply appreciate that Psyche curated this experience for me to fully understand the process I've been living through that hasn't always been easy to articulate.

Willow: Beautiful, yes. A sacred mirror.

Living the Dream Onward

Exactly five years before I wandered Jerusalem in my dreams, I embarked on a different sort of pilgrimage in my waking life. In the summer of 2018, I was invited to attend an artist's residency in a remote mountain village in Southern Crete, where I lived among abandoned ruins and an eclectic group of international composers, painters and poets. There, I was sequestered in the cool cave of my bedroom, chiseled from the mountain's stone, emerging only when the sun descended over the Libyan Sea to wander the narrow alleyways that snaked through the town. The cicadas hummed in a constant chorus, and I felt filled with a sensation I rarely recognized in life: I felt carefree.

Ever since I was a child, I relished my own solitude, and in this waking dreamtime, I moved languidly, the hours unfolding at the pace of my soul. It was in the company of my own aloneness that I experienced a rare and eternal sense of peace. The psychoanalyst, Donald Winnicott, once wrote: "It is a joy to be hidden and a disaster not to be found" (2016, p. 439). In the dream that was that summer, I drifted far, far away like a kite rising into the open sky, trusting that someone or something was holding the spool from which I was flying free.

On my last night in the village, I wandered into the hills as the light faded from pale indigo to lavender. Unlatching heavy gates, I cut across pastures of olive trees, the bells of goats echoing into the distance. It was the last time I recall my body easily carrying me by foot without having to painstakingly calculate the distance, determining if I would have the physical energy to retrace my steps before collapsing from too much exertion.

As night descended, the abandoned habitations felt sinister and disquieting. The wind rattled the loose shutters, an eerie creaking whistling through the maze of pathways up the mountain. I asked the moon to watch over me as I made deliberate strides toward the safe haven of my little abode. I dreamed of ghosts lurking behind the empty window frames, rattling the chains that locked heavy wooden doors, protecting nothing but broken dishware and decaying books. I remember intentionally pausing on the path, facing into fear. Could I befriend this overwhelming dread? Like a precognition, perhaps I sensed it without fully understanding it: the pathway home—the next several years of my life as I would come to know it—would be filled with fear around every corner. I exhaled and put one foot in front of the other.

~~~

I believed the beautiful dream of a Mediterranean summer would overflow indefinitely into my life when I returned home. I had finally secured a position as the counselor at a prestigious school for girls, a role that promised financial stability. I was also falling in love with the man who would become my husband. All seemed poised for security, comfort, and prosperity. I could not have been more wrong.

It began with a tingling in my left arm, the kind of pins and needles sensation when you hit your "funny bone." The sensation seized the nerves on the left side of my face, intermittently paralyzing the connected muscles. Climbing the three flights to my office at the school left me winded and weak. I covertly stole an hour's nap midafternoon to stave off visitations of intense fatigue. I would lock the door, collapse in the armchair, and close my eyes. I knew something was deeply wrong within the marrow of my bones, but how to stop the play of my life without letting down the production and the audience? The private school for girls embodied the cradle of perfection; I, too, felt the need to prove my professional prowess.

One afternoon, a timid girl showed up at the threshold of my office door. Linea had been experiencing panic attacks and as she sat across from me, stunned like a young doe in the headlights, I felt similarly disoriented.[3] Anxiety, perfectionism, disordered eating, my inner clinician ticked off, as she awkwardly relayed her experience. My mind searched for words to respond, but couldn't find them. It was as though every word had been hidden haphazardly in random drawers and every time I opened one, I could see the word but couldn't say it. This girl needs a good therapist, I thought.

And then I realized I was supposed to be that person. To save face, I cut the meeting short, stating she should come back on Thursday and we would take it from there. I gathered up my coat and scarf and tucked my lunch dishes beneath my desk. I'll bring these down to the cafeteria tomorrow, I thought. I locked the door to my office and unbeknownst to me would never return again.

Naively, I assumed that visits to rheumatologists and neurologists would offer straightforward, effective answers: take this pill and proceed with life as planned. But as I entered the gauntlet of encounters with specialists, it was as though I fell down the same rabbit hole as Alice, into a Wonderland where everything was upside down and inside out. Being gaslighted by more than one doctor had a dizzying, de-realizing effect. One neurologist outright told me that "nothing was wrong with me—except that I *thought* something was wrong with me." He prescribed
~~~

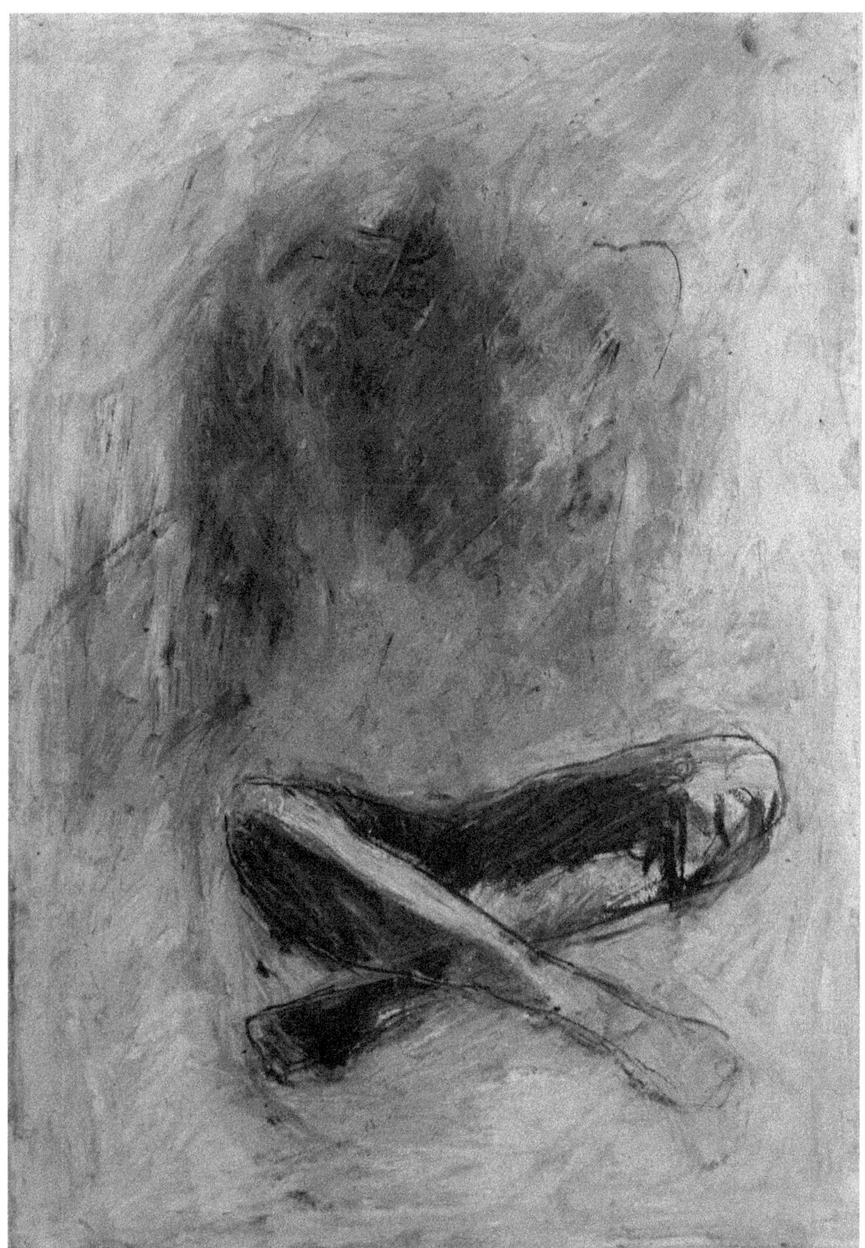

FIGURE 6.1 Figure from *Bodywork* (2024). Oil stick and charcoal on paper.

cognitive-behavioral therapy. Meanwhile, I awoke most mornings feeling as if I had been steamrolled, my limbs filled with lead, the nerves on the left side of my brain and body radiating pain. The sense of volition that had once fueled my professional and social life began to dissolve as I struggled to hold onto some semblance of myself. Fatigue, like quicksand, threatened to pull me further down into an underworld from which I feared I would never emerge.

I frantically and unsuccessfully searched for the escape route in this underworld, and like Alice, I was forced to negotiate characters and phenomena that felt entirely nonsensical, absurd, and frightening. The "real world" began to fuse and transmute into living nightmares. Alice remarks in *Through The Looking Glass* (Carroll, 1882): "A dream is not reality, but who's to say which is which?"

At thirty-four years old, a complex mysterious illness hijacked my immune system, eating at the myelin sheaths that protected my nerves, interrupting the essential messages relayed along those circuits between brain and limbs. I took what I thought would be a short medical leave of absence. But my plan to return for the fall semester was quickly dismantled when I became bed bound. I watched as the hard-earned achievements of my life came to fall like large chunks of ice in a slow-motion avalanche. The belief that through discipline and hard work I could control the outcome of my circumstances, also fractured and crumbled.

"*Enter the beautiful nightmare*." I scribed these words in my journal in 2019. If my life was a nightmare, at least I found it beautiful. I contribute this perspective to a subtle, yet impactful reorientation in my psychology: my ability to be present with my life became more capacious when I approached my days as a series of waking dreams. We often expect our night dreams to be peculiar and disturbing. As a result, it's easier to become curious about their bizarre nature. We know, after all, "it's just a dream." We can explore these strange, surreal worlds aware that the dream will dissipate eventually. In approaching my waking life from the same orientation, I consequently felt less disturbed and more bemused by odd encounters in my medical odyssey. I also learned by necessity how to cope with physical pain garnered with the truth that these sensations, however uncomfortable, were also inherently temporary and ultimately dreamlike.

In his memoir, *In Love with the World*, Yongey Mingyur Rinpoche, the Tibetan Buddhist teacher I referenced in the dream dialogue, writes:

> Dreams are like every other aspect of our existence: They happen, we experience them, but they are not real; their appearance is deceptive, and we easily recognize this non-real aspect of our dreams. This is why dreams are so valuable for understanding the emptiness aspect of reality. Everything is infused with emptiness, and that includes our bodies and our blood, our boulders, our names, and our dreams. To say that life is a dream acknowledges the ceaseless, boundless quality of emptiness in ourselves, in our loved ones, our iPhones, airplanes, food, anger, lust, wealth—in everything. Phenomena have no inherent existence; everything arises from emptiness and never separates from emptiness. Yet

it's a lot easier to perceive this with nighttime dreams than to acknowledge our own emptiness by looking into the mirror.

(Mingyur & Tworkov, 2019, p. 116)

Long-term illness forces one into a nightmarish obstacle course of bureaucracy where insurance companies and the doctors they pay to do evaluations determine the fate of your treatment and access to disability payments. I was subjected to often humiliating questions and tedious assessments. Yet rather than fixate on these indignities and strange encounters as solid and real, I entered into them as waking dreams. A motley cast of characters presented as infusion nurses, phlebotomists, MRI technicians, and insurance bureaucrats. There was Sandra, the social worker who assisted me in my Social Security disability case, and Melanie, the attorney for the hearing. She was well-rehearsed at her script, to the point, efficient, and effective. There was Denis at the California Bureau of Insurance who helped me with my appeal against the health insurance company when they denied paying for a major immune-modulating treatment. I began to see everyone as a dream character, acting their parts. I was surprised to find myself cast in the role of patient.

Like all initiations, the known is irrevocably swept away and exchanged for the unknown. There is no going back to life as it once was. The dream in which my backpack, containing my wallet, my passport, my identification, is stolen announces this initiation: my identity as I have understood it, as I have constructed my life around it, has been taken from me. I am left as a wanderer, stripped of material belongings, forced to live onward, to discover how to exist without the illusions of security I had always relied upon. When I was able to cease frantically grasping for the past I had always known and become curious about this unknown territory, each new scenario did feel oddly dreamlike. Approaching my waking life as though it were a dream, allowed me to feel less anxious and less attached to particular outcomes. I could experience the inherent emptiness of all things as Yongey Mingyur Rinpoche so beautifully describes. I perceived how the seemingly fixed roles of those I met along my medical odyssey were ultimately transparent and flimsy. At any moment, they could dissolve and dissipate. The judge ruling over my disability case someday could fall sick and need disability payments himself. The health insurance bureaucrats could one day have a critical claim of their own denied. The doctor reviewing my case could in the future have some incurable disease and seek treatments that insurance won't pay for. All of these roles eventually will lose their status and meaning. If we are lucky enough to reach old age, we will return to a state of dependence, reliant on the care of others, our bodies subject to disintegration before they ultimately disappear.

Power, as I came to see it, is a temporary illusion that we think keeps us safe.

~~~

Illness wreaked its havoc, and at the center of the debris and rubble, what remained was my inner world. Psyche responded to this "natural disaster" by
~~~

producing a flood of dreams as it tried to make sense of incomprehensible changes. While my outer world shrunk, my inner world, in turn, became richer and more abundant. At night, Psyche's employment worked double-time as she curated images and metaphors and symbols with an ardent, urgent passion. In one dream, *I was trapped in a vehicle, drowning to my demise at the bottom of the ocean.* Another dream, *portended hope as I danced expressively on a stage with an IV pole as my dance partner.* In yet another dream, *I was lost at night in the mountains, the landscape imperceivable, shrouded in shadow, as a voice whispered in my ear: "You are learning to see in the dark."* Once I dreamed *of a creature, part crab, part stork, snapping its jaws and claws at me. Cruelly, I tried to stuff it in a bag. But soon after I realized that the creature was suffering and afraid and needed me to release it into open waters.* Whenever I am overcome with fear, anxiously trying to suppress the illness, I think of the dream creature and soften, eliciting more self-compassion for the parts of me that are afraid.

Our dreams can haunt us as much as they awaken within us new possibilities and emotional truths. Writer and cancer survivor Suleika Jaouad describes the six weeks during her second bone-marrow transplant when she was sequestered to a hospital room "in a kind of sensory deprivation tank, under fluorescent lights, surrounded by so much beige. There was nothing to feast my eyes upon, no visual splendor to lift me up or lighten my days. You can start to lose it when you're locked in a room like that, especially when you're in pain or afraid, which is inevitable in a situation like mine … I ended up with two blood infections and an excruciating combination of kidney issues and mucositis. Since I had a white blood cell count of zero, I knew I could easily die" (Jaouad, 2023).

She goes on to write: "What saved me in those hardest moments was my watercolors. Intuitively I knew that the only way to keep from losing faith or losing my mind was to engage with the brutal realities I was facing—everything from the physical objects like hospitals gowns and wheelchairs to the existential questions that arise when facing one's own imminent mortality. But I couldn't do it head-on. I needed to see the truth but see it slant … It felt safer and more productive to engage with it on a symbolic level—what the writer Joseph Campbell calls the 'mythopoetic.'"

She describes a permeability between her conscious and unconscious mind, partially due to high doses of medications and resultant fever dreams. What emerges, to her own surprise, is a series of watercolor paintings: "Take the first painting I made, where I'm in my hospital bed … nestled in a tree just outside the window, overlooking the city's nightscape. In another, I'm standing on a watermelon, with an elephant on its hind legs as my IV pole: a very precarious balancing act. In still another, I'm a half human, half sea creature in dark blue water. Though I love swimming, I'm terrified when I can't see the bottom; I panic if the slightest bit of seaweed touches my foot. And yet there I am in the deep, descending even deeper amid all these creatures. Rendering my medical situation in these different landscapes and locales was a way to acknowledge my immediate reality, but also to make room for other possibilities. It only occurs to me now that in these paintings, I was establishing a visual language for holding both hardship and hope in one palm."

Psyche communicates through images in waking or sleeping dreams, or some state in between. When trapped in a body with an immune system revolting, confined to the cell of a hospital room, dreams and imagery, as Jaouad so poignantly describes, offer a mythical world beyond one's imminent reality. The limitations of an individual's condition no longer apply in the realm of dreams.

Everything is moveable and capable of metamorphosis.

In 2018, I was diagnosed with myalgic encephalomyelitis, also known as Chronic Fatigue Syndrome. In my waking life at that time, I could barely walk around the block or stand in the shower due to muscular weakness and shortness of breath, but in my sleeping dreams, *I could swim effortlessly for miles upon miles down an ebony river glittering with the night's stars.* In my dreams, *I often danced with abandon, never tiring; I ascended mountains, trekked across plateaus, and viscerally remembered my vitality.* Like Jaouad, my dreams offered up an abundance of metaphors, amplifying my worst fears and my most ardent hopes.

While in waking life disabilities dictate what is and isn't possible, in sleeping dreams, these rules do not apply. People with acquired blindness, for example, report still being able to dream in visual images. Their brain has the ability to draw on visual memories thanks to related brain circuits that were formed before the onset of blindness.

No matter how dire our circumstances, we can always experience liberation through dreaming. A study based on the testimonies of former Auschwitz concentration camp prisoners to Polish psychiatrists in 1973 illuminates a collective practice of dream interpretation.

> The custom of interpreting dreams in Auschwitz can be described as a complex and multilevel ritual that had at least three dimensions: individual, interpersonal, and social. On the individual level, this ritual was oriented on revealing the inmates' future. A prisoner, listening to a dream reader, could receive a good or bad prophecy, and this uncertainty was the core of the process. The interpersonal dimension of this ritual was connected with the inmates' need to capture others' attention. On the social level, dream sharing was a community-building activity. On each of these levels, finding the meaning of a dream was not as important as being engaged in closer relationships with other inmates.
>
> (Owczarski, 2017)

Invoking dreams collectively helped prisoners to exist in an imaginal realm that transcended the horror of their daily experience in the concentration camp.

Our dream lives can offer a portal to liberation, a play-space for our deepest desires, a counterpoint to the brutal and sometimes devastating traumas of cultural, historical forces. Jonathan W. White, American Civil War historian, studied around four-hundred dreams of soldiers and prisoners as he discovered their descriptions in personal memoirs, letters, and diaries. The savage conditions for captured fighters in the Civil War had them living in deep squalor. Forced to bury fellow prisoners who died of starvation, prisoners were constantly exposed to disease and often ill.

But in their dreams, they could travel far away from all that. In her review of White's book, *Midnight in America: Darkness, Sleep and Dreams During the Civil War,* Sarah Kershaw writes:

> It was only in their sleep, in their unconscious minds, that the prisoners of war were free, making an ethereal escape from their wretched reality … Some dreamed of escape. Some dreamed of death. Some dreamed of survival. Some dreamed of beef and oysters, buffets and banquets. Some dreamed of kissing their wives and sweethearts. Some dreamed their women were unfaithful. Some dreamed of giant lice. Many dreamed of home.
>
> (Kershaw, 2021)

White furthers this notion: "Dreams, for many of them, played a comforting role … The most common dreams soldiers had were of home, hugging or kissing their wives, picking up their children" (Kershaw, 2021). He also learned that Civil War prisoners, mirroring the study of inmates at Auschwitz, found psychological resilience and fortitude in sharing their dreams with each other.

The practice of entrusting our dream lives to a confidant benefits not only the dreamer but also the listener. Too often, we view our dreams as "crazy" or "random," casting them off into the shadows as we move into the light and go about our days. Neglected, the potential insights of our dreams wither away. Knowing that I had the opportunity to bring a dream to Willow to tend together, I became a more sensitive, inquisitive receptor. I paid careful attention to Psyche's communications, writing down her images in a state of wonder. Often at the end of our dream sessions, the listener remarked that she, too, felt transformed by the dream. We embarked on a shared invitation into reverie. Multiple meanings became amplified through co-exploration. What was once just my dream or Willow's dream, now lives intrapsychically in both of us.

A contemporary study of a dream group run by a seasoned social worker at a women's maximum-security prison in South Carolina, exemplifies how dreams, when tended in a safe and respectful container, transform not just the dreamer, but also the group as a whole. The incarcerated women who participated in the group often expressed feelings of powerlessness due to their past traumas, victimization, and current withdrawals of everyday freedoms. The social worker facilitating the dream group invited each participant to make the presented dream her own: members were encouraged to share their own feelings that they associated with the dream, the intention being to create a collage of meanings that may be helpful to the dreamer. The dreamer, in turn, responded with her own associations.

Not surprisingly, many of the women suffered from regular nightmares. Engaging in dreamwork helped them to "gain a sense of mastery amidst so many feelings of powerlessness in prison" (DeHart, 2005, p. 15). One woman reflected: "[I like] rewriting the dreams. I learned how to give a better ending to dreams. I can take power away from my nightmares, take power back." They also learned the practice of imaginal dialogue so that they could deepen their relationship to certain dream symbols or images. One woman described: "If you wanted to find out more about your dream, the dream is an extension of yourself, so you can have a dialogue with yourself or whoever was in your dream to find out more."

This brings to mind a quote from Eckhart Tolle (2010): "When you are trapped in a nightmare, your motivation to awaken will be so much greater than that of someone caught up in a relatively pleasant dream." The group container catalyzed unusually intimate and deep connections between members through revelation, nonjudgmental reflection, and curiosity in a harsh prison environment typically necessitating strong defenses. Communal dream practice allowed the participants to express their vulnerability, shame, fears, and hopes, and to feel honored and held by the other group members. Women reported gaining new insights into themselves, their past traumas and crimes, as well as experiencing enhanced physical and emotional wellbeing and renewed hope for their future. On an interpersonal level, women attributed the group to growing more meaningful relationships with fellow inmates as they learned to appreciate others' perspectives. The study concluded that the dream group fostered self-awareness and the cultivation of introspection. Intrapsychically and interpersonally, the inmates evolved their relationships to self and other more consciously and creatively.

~~~

Even as our bodies may be entrapped by illness, imprisonment, war, disability, or our own minds, Psyche offers a phenomenal gift: an infinite portal to endless freedom through our dreams. During my own odyssey with mysterious long-term illness, my dream life overflowed with images. Some dreams were thematic of hope—mixing shades of luscious green as I painted new leaves budding from a plant—and other dreams portended fears of my own demise and disintegration. Yet, even nightmares offered me new metaphors for understanding my complex grief, longings, and losses. I am forever grateful to the enigmatic ways of Psyche as she spins her artistry. Without her creations, my life would have been flattened to the often dire, depressing circumstances I faced. Yet with Psyche's companionship, I experienced possibility and potential, the raw transformative materials of creativity. My reverence for Psyche grew a thousandfold as she helped me to make meaning of wildly confounding and unchosen changes. During the numerous physical hardships and psychological struggles of those years, Psyche's creativity was not only a lifeline, but a lifesaver.
~~~

Notes

1 It's salient to note that I experienced this dream in 2023, prior to October 7, 2023, so my associations with Israel did not include the terrorist attack by Hamas and the ensuing violence, war, and humanitarian crisis.
2 For a wonderful dissertation on illness dreams, see Beauchene (2025).
3 To protect client confidentiality, I am using a pseudonym and changing some client details while staying true to the essence of the presenting issues.

References

Beauchene, K. M. (2025). *Illness dreams: Interpreting clinical approaches from Greek antiquity to modernity* (Order No. 32122148) [Doctoral Dissertation, Pacific Graduate Institute]. Dissertations & Theses @ Pacifica Graduate Institute. https://www.proquest.com/dissertations-theses/illness-dreams-interpreting-clinical-approaches/docview/3228594628/se-2

Carroll, L. (1882). *Through the looking glass, and what Alice found there*. Macmillan & Co.

DeHart, D. (2005). Cognitive restructuring through dreams & imagery: Descriptive analysis of a women's prison-based program. *Journal of Offender Rehabilitation, 49*(1), 23–38.

Jaouad, S. (2023). Prompt 240: A new way to see. *The Isolation Journals*. https://substack.com/@theisolationjournals

Kershaw, S. (2021, October 27). How prisoners of war used their dreams to help them survive. *Washington Post*. https://www.washingtonpost.com/news/inspired-life/wp/2015/11/05/how-prisoners-of-war-used-their-dreams-to-help-them-survive/

Leonard, E. T. (2024). *Bodywork*. Bored Wolves and Firehouse Press.

Mingyur, Y., & Tworkov, H. (2019). *In love with the world: A monk's journey through the bardos of living and dying*. Random House.

Owczarski, W. (2017). The ritual of dream interpretation in the Auschwitz concentration camp. *Dreaming, 27*(4), 278–289. https://doi.org/10.1037/drm0000064

Tolle, E. (2010). An Interview with Eckhart Tolle: The power of now and the end of suffering [Excerpt]. *The TAT Forum*. (Original work from Sounds True in 2008.)

Winnicott, D. W. (2016). Communicating and not communicating leading to a study of opposites. In L. Caldwell & H. T. Robinson (Eds.), *The collected works of D. W. Winnicott, Vol. 6 (1960–1963)* (pp. 433–446). Oxford University Press.

Zweig, C. (2021). *The inner work of age: Shifting from role to soul*. Park Street Press.

7

WANTING OUT

Learning from Cats—Bardo and the Shoji Screen

I was mortally terrified that my beloved cat Bardo[1] would escape from my new loft, so I bought a three-sided shoji screen to seal off the front entrance. It has worked really well. It makes a little space between the front door and the living space inside of my home in which to ensure that Bardo does not escape.

But she doesn't appreciate this protective seal, this barrier to the great beyond. Every few days she begins to howl her complaint and pace back and forth by the screen or even occasionally to scale the shoji screen in defiance. A couple of times, she has even climbed over the shoji screen into the gap between the front door and the screen. An indoor cat who tasted the life of the outdoors as a young mother (she was rescued in a church with her three kittens), her innate wildness must declare itself every so often and push past the bounds of domesticity to claim her total aliveness. Even if it means she might be destroyed. We both know this. So although I do chastise her and voice a firm "No!" and so signal and define the necessary limits of acceptable behavior, and although she does heed this warning signal for a spell, we both know that eventually her need to rebel will return for another round of protest.

Her wail is no mere plaintive cry. It is a soul-wrenching, gut-clenching howl. A cat howl. Most people think of a dog howl when they think of a howl, but when you live with cats whom you are madly in love with, you are deeply attuned to the feline howl. It's excruciating to hear—especially when I know that I could let her out if I really wanted to. But I do not dare risk losing her, my most precious little girl.

Yet, her howl wrecks me. I resonate with the magnetizing pull of the great beyond.

Michael Eigen (2018) calls this "TIP: The Impossible Place." Like Bardo, I imagine that once I am on the other side of the shoji screen I will somehow know true liberation, freedom, and finally see God and make direct contact. What The Impossible Place helps me to discover, when I hold it as such, is that I am always

DOI: 10.4324/9781003591863-8

already on the other side of the shoji screen, from the reverse perspective. I have already broken through to the other side, and it is where I live.

From this perspective, I am already found. Already free. Already united with God. And this is what it's like. It's like being separated from God, yearning for a liberation I imagine that I don't already have, which, ironically, can be freeing. Until the perspective from behind the shoji screen reverses again and I fail to see its double-sided nature.

In rare moments, the shoji screen opens up in my imagination, and I can experience both sides at once. From this place, Bardo is free to come and go without restraint. That is the place I reach for in what will be our infinite dance of her asking to be let out and my saying, "No baby girl! I'm sorry, I know how much you want to go outside. But it's just not safe out there for you, and I love you too much to let you get hurt."

Our veterinarian's assessment and pronouncement of Bardo's stage three kidney disease now makes clear the double-sidedness of protection and surrender. As I daily administer Bardo's medicine, to help ease her hypertension and slow the inevitable progression of her kidney disease, I am present with the boundless love between us, even as I touch the edges of her near-term disappearance. She will, in time, make her way to the great beyond. No shoji screen can keep death out of reach. Her spirit will break free from her tiny body, from her everyday gray fur coat. We will be separated. Still, tending our sacred bond, through the protection of the inner sanctum of our home, is a path of that very freedom through the lived inseparability of transcendence and immanence.

Opening the Shoji Screen

Eva: There is something about "The Impossible Place" …

Willow: Yes, I think that is what Bardo teaches me about, TIP, The Impossible Place, the way we live it together (Eigen, 2018, pp. 93–105): I'm not willing to fully grant her the freedom of an outdoor cat because of my concern for her safety. And yet I recognize that I can't spare her from death. I can't hold on to her forever, even as I can recognize an eternal bond between us. I can't spare her or me the loss of her.

Eva: Yes. We don't know what animals understand about their finiteness. I don't know if they can conceive of things existentially in the ways that we can, although wild animals have likely encountered death. Who knows if they also understand that "this too will happen to me." We know certain animals do grieve their kin. We can suspect you're holding this knowledge of impermanence in ways that Bardo can't, which is so bittersweet, because Bardo is very much in the moment of "I want out right now," but you're holding a greater understanding of life and death and danger and safety. It's this beautifully excruciating kind of compassion because it means holding this limit out of protection, which I imagine is the hard work of parenting—saying no even when the desire is very much a yes. I'm very touched by your understanding of the time-bounded nature of your relationship with Bardo, which Bardo likely can't conceive. Can you further elaborate on The Impossible Place and what it connotes for you?

Willow: Eigen's phraseology of naming, designating such a psychic space or occasion helps me.

Eva: A word that shows up for me is that which is *unresolvable*, and I would like to understand more of what he meant.

Willow: I think you named it precisely. In giving us, in language, a designation, *T-I-P*, The Impossible Place—the irreconcilable, the unresolvable—Eigen is, in some ways, taking us to the very heart of being and also the heart of psychotherapeutic practice from a psychoanalytic vantage. It's not our job to try to solve a problem. It's our job to try to learn to be with the patient, with the client, to learn from experience with them, which is very much the essence of Bion's teaching, which is in the lineage of Eigen and beyond.

And this prelude that our entire book is woven around—this phrase of "learning from …," learning from life, learning from experience—was Bion's offering of the core of psychoanalytic psychotherapy, about learning from experience rather than trying to solve a problem or fix something. Actually, it's about companioning the client or patient so that we can be curious and learn together as they're facing what they're up against and how they're living that experience. And that we learn that by living TIP with them, in moments, in what Eigen calls Living Moments, which is the title of that first book in 2015 that Stephen Bloch and Loray Daws edited as a Festschrift honoring Michael Eigen.

Eva: It is such a different orientation, the learning with, the learning from, the walking together, acknowledging those places that perhaps are unresolvable. But how do you live with that? My own psychotherapist recently said to me that some grief is unresolvable, and it *should be* actually. And that really felt very surprising to receive in a way because I think in Western paradigms it's often about how you get over something, how you move on, or how you transcend a problem. Certain grief, from a genocide, for example, *should* be unresolvable because we need to know the depth of the impact so that we don't repeat the same horror and atrocity.

And I think there's something very humbling about de-positioning ourselves as psychotherapists from the expert who knows the direction that something's supposed to take, or we somehow have special knowledge about what should and shouldn't happen. But the *companioning with* is a powerful modeling of being with what is irreconcilable or being with what is full of paradox, which is so much of life …

Willow: In terms of paradox, I think about the call to publish this book on sharing our dreams—to engage dream life in this written mode—whereas from many cultural perspectives, including certain indigenous perspectives that I align with, dreams are meant to be handed down in the oral tradition to be safe kept, heart-to-heart, soul-to-soul, and transmitted person to person.

I consider the part of me that honors those concerns. I think this aspect is part of my deep appreciation for engaging the process of this book with you, heart-to-heart, soul-to-soul, psyche-to-psyche in our dialogues. And I hope that in this complicated world that is a hybrid world of multiple cultural identities, the act of communicating through the written word can be a complementary vehicle of meaningful dream sharing and communication. I truly wish that the emotional truth of our dreams in this book can be shared both in writing and orally, just as our dream dialogues themselves have been a hybrid of oral and written communication.

Eva: It's a vulnerable enterprise that we're engaging in. The work is full of revelations, and many of those revelations are quite subtle, exposing even. I am really looking forward to further conversations about these dream dialogues, in our own voices, because I think that will bring alive the emotive experience that you can't necessarily capture just through the written word alone. I'm listening to someone's memoir right now in her own voice, the author's voice. You can't deny somebody's lived experience when it's in their own voice because it's just so intimate.

Willow: I'm glad that we will do both.

Note

1 I named my beloved gray Abyssinian tabby cat "Bardo," not after the actress and sex symbol and animal rights activist Bridgette Bardo as some friends have mused aloud, but rather to invoke and bring me into direct, intimate contemplation-through-relationship with the Buddhist realms of existence: before birth, birth, this life, death, after death, and rebirth. These realms, these bardos, may all be regarded as dreams.

References

Bloch, S., & Daws, L., (Eds.). (2015). *Living moments: On the work of Michael Eigen*. Routledge.

Eigen, M. (2018). *The challenge of being human*. Routledge.

8

CIRCLE GAME

Learning from Cats—Chief and His Exercise Wheel

Here we witness the circle of life through a cat running on his exercise wheel. This simple beholding of a cat expressing his playful aliveness and, later in life, his "going on being," becomes one of turning toward grace in all her mystery. At first, watching him is like a dizzy spell. Then he hits his stride in a steady hum, flying in the sky, even as the ground disappears beneath his paws, his feline body indigenous to the motion of stillness.

Dreaming Chief and His Circle Game

When Chief, my beloved Abyssinian cat, was in his youth, he raced on his exercise wheel like a flying tiger, dressed in his beautiful orange tabby coat. The steady hum of the rotating plastic frame sounded against the bumpers beneath that held the wheel in place, a reverberation created by his circumambulation. To behold Chief was to imagine there was no end in sight to his exuberant energy. Indeed, I had first bought the wheel for Chief in his adolescence because as an indoor tom cat, without the pleasures and perils of the outdoors, he had a lot of energy he needed to expend.

Watching him was *almost* pure joy. I could feel not only his initial exuberance and bliss but also, as his exuberance inevitably waned, *sometimes* his peaceful calm, transmitted through the rhythm of his ride on the black-coated leopard print wheel. Yet, more often, I sensed his unmistakable standstill frustration with simply going round and round. Those were the cycles of his youth.

Now a senior cat, Chief embodies in his distinctively feline ways what psychoanalyst and pediatrician Donald Winnicott referred to in his observation of humans as "going on being." Chief only occasionally gets on his exercise wheel now—and not in the middle of the night as he did in his youth—but every few days, at the very

DOI: 10.4324/9781003591863-9

end of the daylight hours, just before nightfall, as if wanting to extend time and to magnetize and prolong the focus of my attention on him.

He no longer runs for minutes at a clip. Now he just hops on for a minute or two, to walk or trot a few steps only, pausing between tentative jaunts. He yowls to vocalize his pleasure and his angst, mixed together in a call to please me with his demonstration and to voice his frustration at once, a call and response to receive my verbal encouragement and support. "Good boy," I coax and croon, in what is now a part of my sequenced patterned responses to him, suggesting with wide eyes and a nodding head and a minimally encouraging addendum of "mm hmm" that he continue to run the wheel.

In his old age, Chief now accompanies his occasional short-lived running of the wheel with his yowling. In his youth, he was stealth and silent as he flew on his wheel. Now in his elderhood, his progressive, repetitive yowls are as if to remark, "I can't go on. I don't want to go on. I am going on. Watch me go!" And, no sooner has he shifted from a few halting trots into a few steady rounds of jog, before he stops abruptly, commenting with a final yowl, "I'm done." This lamentation in multiple verses of yowl signals to us both that his dream life is gently, almost imperceptibly, according to an unknown window of time and not without the exercise of joy and sorrow bound together, winding to a close.

To amplify recognition of this seasonality of life, this chapter title invokes the song title "Circle Game," written by the great singer Joni Mitchel, a song that I grew up singing and performing.

Purring the Dream

Willow: So Chief is lying down next to the computer with his head on my hand purring away. I don't know if you can hear him …

Eva: I can hear him … Willow, can you speak to the "Circle Game" link?

Willow: Yes, the song "Circle Game," written by the great singer songwriter Joni Mitchell, is a song that I sang twice for my late brother, Scott Pearson, once on stage when we were both in high school, me singing to him while he was in the audience with our whole school, and once upon his death, at fifty years old, for his celebration of life, which was on Zoom at the commencement of COVID.

Eva: Thank you.

Willow: So that's my dream of Chief running his exercise wheel. It's a repetitive waking dream that has been recursive in the ways I describe over the last twelve-and-a-half years that I've had Chief.

Eva: I'm really glad that you're including the more-than-human world in these two chapters on cats because I think it's not just about your dream of Chief, but also Chief's dream of you. As an indoor cat, his entire world is a world that you've created for him, including this wheel for him to express his energy and his will for life. It is so important for readers to know what a powerful cat he is. He's not a regular little house cat. And I can hear that powerful energy now, through his purring as you were reading; that's how deep and resonant it is. I think we develop these very soulful relationships with our animal companions. They become part of our waking and sleeping dreams.

Whether I'm dreaming of a domestic animal companion or dreaming of a fierce animal like a bear or a tiger in the wild—these animal instincts become part of us. Chief's instincts are a part of you. And I think there's something about this animism that is so vital.

In so many traditions, there is an animistic sense that everything is alive and that we are in reciprocity with this aliveness. There isn't a duality. You've formed this deeply soulful relationship with Chief: both of you are dreaming each other at all times, whether it's in your waking dreams or your sleeping dreams. His world is created by you because he doesn't venture out into the urban fray, which is probably a good thing for his safety.

I'm sure if we could know what he dreams of as he sleeps, that you are central in those dreams, and certainly you're central in his waking dreams. And it can be easy to forget that as humans, we're not the only ones who are dreaming. It's meaningful to deposition ourselves as the central characters of our dreams or as the one who is dreaming.

There are owls, deer, foxes, and hawks and so many animals that I share this land with, and they're also having a dream that sometimes might include me and sometimes might not. Yet I do sometimes wonder—when I gaze into the eyes of a deer—what is the dream that they're having of me? So shifting those perspectives around is important in our interpenetration of this existence where the animate world is very much alive and dreaming alongside us.

Willow: We are indeed dreaming one another.

Eva: The part about "going on being,"[1] which sounds like a lyric from a blues song, speaks to how life is full of pleasure and angst simultaneously. You captured that tension between Chief's desire to go on, but also the lamentation of aging. I wonder if you can say more about what "going on being" means to you?

Willow: It's complicated for Chief at his age, and what I am aware of is that at thirteen, he's made a turn toward descent; he's no longer in his rising. And we could say his present descent will one day transition to an ascent that's apart from his rising into this worldly life. There is a way in which he's struggling with being here now, in a way that he hasn't struggled until just the past couple of years. And I feel his struggle. We're both being with that struggle together, and it is most emblematic—it is most brought to bear—in his patterning on his exercise wheel as I've described. His struggle gets vividly embodied, that tension between volition and surrender and giving up and allowing.

Eva: I'm thinking of the Buddhist Wheel of Life …

Willow: Yes, the Dharma Wheel, the wheel of truth …

Eva: Yes, the Dharma Wheel. How many beautiful depictions there are of that image, and what it means to jump off the wheel, liberated from continuous reincarnation. To jump off would mean you are enlightened?

Willow: I think some would say that the enlightened action would be to continue.

Eva: Right, as a bodhisattva, to return and help sentient beings reach enlightenment as well, or the end of suffering.

Willow: Again and again and again.

Eva: Going round and round on the wheel perpetually is painstakingly hard. It is full of challenge and difficulty, beauty and revelation. I fantasize how liberating it would be to finally jump off the wheel and be free! I feel vicarious relief when Chief leaps off his exercise wheel! The "Circle Game," the Dharma Wheel, and Chief's Exercise Wheel, all blend together for me. I was really touched by your invocation of your singing the "Circle Game" at your brother Scott's celebration of life. It brought tears to my eyes because it's such a beautiful song. I wept the first time I heard it as a child; I understood the transmission of that song even as a little person in the world with very little life experience.

Willow: Yes, we do revolve on the Dharmic Wheel of Life, and we never know when suddenly we might be pushed off the wheel and it *is* the "Circle Game." We don't know what season is next.

By the way, as we're talking, Chief has his head pressed against my hand. He's very much a part of this conversation.

Eva: This is the first time he has joined us.

Willow: Yes, it is the first time in our years of dream dialogues that he is joining our conversation.

Eva: Which is quite remarkable, actually. I didn't know that he even came up the stairs into your office.

Willow: He preceded me up the loft stairs on my way to this conversation. And as I say, he was a little bit uncontainable a few moments ago. He was pacing across the computer before we began.

Eva: That's so interesting.

Willow: I think there's something vitally important about how our animal companions involve us in what my dear friend and colleague Stephen Bloch and I have been calling the "primal transcendent,"[2] meaning how the instinctual realm is none other than the vibrantly, dynamically embodied transcendent. And my dream of Chief and his dream with me is a constancy of that primal transcendent, of that instinctual immanence that is never other than this *real* illusory dream nature.

Eva: That's a very powerful phrase: primal being of the earth, immanent being of the now, and transcendent being of the spirit. Our soulful relationships with our animal companions are on the one hand very tactile, direct and primal; on the other hand, the bond between souls transcends language.

Willow: Yes, I certainly experience my relationship with my feline companions as some of the most intimate relationships of my life. As many people do. The emotional bond, the emotional truth of our bond, is ... the nature of the *primal transcendent* directly, literally in touch with that transcendence where spirit and substance are not two.

Notes

1 This refers to pediatrician and psychoanalyst D. W. Winnicott's phrase about sourcing the will of psychic life.

2 See forthcoming chapter, "How Music Dreams the 'Hum' of a Session: Stephen Bloch and Willow Pearson Trimbach in Conversation" In forthcoming publication by S. Bloch and W. Pearson Trimbach, *The Ear of the Heart: Music, Psyche, Transcendence and Immanence*.

9

DEVOTION

Learning from Nondual Love

This chapter centers on dreams of four of my principal teachers. Each teacher guided my formal spiritual practice, through the Buddhist path of meditation, joined with the study and application of transpersonal, integral, and psychoanalytic psychotherapy. For context, in 1996, I entered the master's program in Transpersonal Counseling Psychology (TCP) with a concentration in music therapy at Naropa University,[1] a Buddhist-inspired university. A deep artery through the heart of my training at Naropa was meditation, specifically the following forms of meditation in the Tibetan Buddhist tradition: shamatha (calm abiding), vipassana (insight), and tonglen (compassionate exchange, or taking and sending). I thank Dale Asrael[2] for transmission of and instruction in these skillful means of spiritual practice, taught in the context of transpersonal psychotherapy training, which constitutes the groundwater of my clinical work.

During and following my years of training in psychotherapy, meditation, and music therapy at Naropa, I collaborated, studied, practiced, and taught with integral philosopher Ken Wilber[3] from 1996–2008. Ken Wilber is an integral theorist and author of more than twenty books that apply his integral vision to all domains of human knowledge. His past teaching activity through the founding of the Integral Institute and his current influence through the online media presence of Integral Life has catalyzed and inspired a worldwide community of integral scholar-practitioners. Ken is a complex character, long evoking deep regard and deep critique, in equally conflictual measure, on an international level.

In collaborating with and learning from Ken through the Integral Institute, I was deeply inspired by his vision of human potential. As his student, I began to ask, in my twenties, what is Mahamudra? What is nonduality? I had no idea. But I had a taste for the yet unknown communications that these honored words seemed to hold open and invite.

DOI: 10.4324/9781003591863-10

Through the in-person Integral Institute seminars, created in concert with Ken, I received the life lesson that we are all transmitting our states of being to one another 24/7. Through Ken's teaching, I came to appreciate the power, the light, and the shadow of conceptual thought to variously inspire, pursue, approach, invoke, and transmit psychospiritual practice. For more than twelve years, I learned, taught, wrote about, and applied Ken's integral frameworks, which continue to inform my creative scholarship, teaching, and practice today.

In 2006, inspired by the call of Mahamudra and nonduality that Naropa University and Ken Wilber had introduced, I entered American Buddhist teacher Lama Palden's[4] six-year lineage program at Sukhasiddi Foundation.[5] Sukhasiddhi Foundation is a Buddhist center in Northern California's San Francisco Bay Area. It was created and is stewarded by Lama Palden. The center is rooted in the teachings of two fully awakened women, Sukhasiddhi and Niguma. Sukhasiddhi Foundation guides its students in the Shangpa and Kagyu lineages of Tibetan Buddhism in America. This lineage program that Lama Palden teaches brings the traditional three-year Buddhist retreat to laypeople.

Taking formal refuge vows with Lama Palden, who is much beloved as a realized yogini and transmitter of the authentic Buddhadharma in the West, I engaged Vajrayana and Mahamudra practice through this lineage program. Through Lama Palden's example, I came to appreciate living Buddha nature, as both a woman and as an American woman. Her teachings provided the ground from which, with her cross-cultural translations, I was able to approach my root teacher Khenpo Tsültrim Gyamtso Rinpoche, who was Tibetan. Without her kind guidance, I would not have been able to make a meaningful connection to or absorb the mandala of teachings that Rinpoche initiated. An ongoing deepening of contemplative being, flowing from her instruction, infuses the ground and practice of all aspects of my work.

I entered the program at Sukhasiddi in tandem with approaching and commencing study and practice with Buddhist master Khenpo Tsültrim Gyamtso Rinpoche.[6] Khenpo Tsültrim Gyamtso Rinpoche was a Tibetan Buddhist master of the highest order of scholarship, practice, realization, and transmission, who devoted his life to teaching the Buddhadharma internationally. Long regarded worldwide as a Buddha of the twenty-first century, he founded several nunneries, including in Bhutan and Nepal.[7] His inconceivable teaching activity is a blessing that continues to shine across the globe.

I approached Khenpo Tsültrim Gyamtso Rinpoche in 2005, seeking his instruction. Through a combination of in-person teachings, service, teachings by video, and intensive practice, I learned from Rinpoche the equality of samsara and nirvana as the dawning of Mahamudra through guru yoga. In particular, through Rinpoche, I came to the path of essence, as nada yoga, through hearing, studying, and singing songs of realization and the transmission of sound–emptiness–sound.

Expressly, through Rinpoche, the practice of dream yoga, the illusion-like true nature of being, continues to dawn and became the basis of this book. Learning from Rinpoche, through the Marpa Foundation,[8] was greatly supported by his American disciples and translators Ari and Rose Goldfield,[9] together with the teaching activity of his Tibetan disciple Dzogchen Ponlop Rinpoche,[10] founder of Nalandabodhi Seattle.[11]

My efforts to integrate this dedicated spiritual practice, across these interwoven and yet distinct mandalas, led me to study psychoanalytic psychotherapy at the Wright Institute in Berkeley, California, where I encountered the resonant writings of psychoanalysts James Grotstein[12] and Michael Eigen.[13] I approached Dr. Grotstein for theoretical and clinical consultation, receiving his generous mentorship in the last few years of his life. Then, upon his death, I was fortunate to enter the Michael Eigen workshop mandala—the international sphere of communication among a dedicated group of Eigen's students—by the grace of an invitation from dear colleague and friend, psychologist Robin Bagai.[14]

Michael Eigen, a psychologist and psychoanalyst, is the author of more than thirty books. He teaches through New York University's Postdoctoral Program in Psychotherapy and Psychoanalysis and conducts an international seminar, now online, on the work of psychoanalyst Wilfred Bion and his own work. Eigen is quietly heralded among scholar clinicians as a renegade and revolutionary at the leading edge of psychoanalysis.

I came to study with Dr. Eigen, initially through his online listserv in 2014. Over the decade plus that I have engaged in study as a part of the Eigen mandala—through the listserv, his seminars, in applying his work clinically, teaching his work to my students at the California Institute of Integral Studies, and writing about its impact—I have learned something more about our humanity and our capacity for *psychic democracy*[15] (equally welcoming of our young, our playful, and our mature, thoughtful dimensions of being, together with our obstructing dimensions). I have also come to appreciate the unending nature of opening to experience, inseparable from the coemergent pain and beauty of life. Through Dr. Eigen, I have come to appreciate the wisdom of working with suffering *a bit at a time*. Not trying to escape it. *Not trying to do too much.* Helped by his teaching, dreaming a psychotherapy session is now vivid, in the sense of realizing all communication between client and therapist, and the therapist's correspondent reverie, as waking dream thoughts and feelings. Through working with Dr. Eigen's teaching, I have more humility in the face of seeming opposites—majesty and catastrophe. Through the Eigen mandala, I continue to welcome our *artistry of the invisible* (Masih, 2021). Dr. Eigen, by his example, welcomes a spirit of play; I find myself sourcing a deeper spirit of play in psychotherapy and in teaching, now composing a trinity of regard for love, work, and play, in concert.

Receiving these combined teachings, through these nested mandalas of awakening, invites me to now receive my students, patients, family, friends, cats, strangers, and world as dream teachers. The teaching is unending. The learning is unending. An equality of meditation and post-meditation as pure being continues to open up. An equality of non-conceptuality and conceptuality, an equality of preferences and equal taste, opens further.

Now a one-pointed path of essence, dreaming guides my way.

And I return to where I started, singing a little dream mantra that wakes me up, inhaling and exhaling: "Free the Many, find the One; taste the Many as the One."

Through my practice with these teachers, I have received, discovered, and continue to learn from *nondual love*, born of the heart of dream devotion.[16] *Nondual love* is a term that can be defined as boundless, immeasurable, ever-evolving love, aspiring to recognize and behold all beings—including ourselves—in all states and all stages of wisdom and confusion.

These ever-nested mandalas—integral, Buddhist, psychotherapeutic/psychoanalytic, mystic, artistic—quicken us, as participants, to awakening, through our collective wisdom and confusion. I am grateful to be held by and to contribute to these collective communities.[17]

As we all do, I came to study with each of my root teachers, key mentors situated at the center of each of these mandalas, during different developmental eras in my life. As such, my own desires, gifts, and yearnings—my own flavors of wisdom and confusion—differently, distinctly, and variously catalyzed, impeded, and furthered my learning from and with each of them. By their grace, I was invited to learn something of their wisdom; as happens by the grace of living the genuine teachings, I continue to learn according to the wisdom *and* the confusion encountered, just as my students and my patients do with me. Through this nondual love, I am held in the creative unknown, now extending this nondual love through my own being. The collective background presence of these four principal teachers is no less than enlightening.

What I am most grateful for is how, by internalizing each of them in all that I am able to appreciate of their complexity (which is necessarily and inevitably a limited understanding of who they each are), each of these root mentors continues to teach me through the practice of dream yoga. In my experience, their combined instruction has coalesced as the path of essence, through the practice of dreaming, a practice of waking up to genuine reality.

Dreaming Khenpo Tsültrim Gyamtso Rinpoche (KTGR)

This dream visited me on January 20, 2024. Khenpo Tsültrim Gyamtso Rinpoche (KTGR),[18] my root teacher, died on June 22, 2024, at ninety years old.

> *I dream of Rinpoche. He is at the door. I sit next to him (he is on my left) as I answer the test, the oral exam. Someone else is asking me the questions and KTGR is evaluating my response.*
>
> *I take Jamie's car to Los Angeles and call her to ask how to put gas in her car. She tells me over the phone that I need to connect with her mechanic.*
>
> *I am on the on ramp, and Tim, in a silver Honda, comes by. His car is a near miss.*

Sarah and Mary arrive at the door to help me translate. Rinpoche retreats, yet I introduce them to Rinpoche, who talks to them in English.

I go to the bathroom before dinner.

I sit next to Rinpoche and demonstrate my noticing of his soft, subtle brush of my left side, by turning toward him and smiling, without anyone else noticing.

I am offered up to three months housing for becoming a translator. I think that becoming a translator is the best life path I can imagine pursuing.

Eva and Willow: Apprenticing the Dream

Eva: What was the emotional flavor of the dream upon waking?

Willow: I had a sense of profound gratitude, to experience direct connection to my teacher in this way. And also reassurance.

Eva: Yes, I felt that in terms of the soft, subtle brush, the knowing smile, and glance that's shared just between the two of you. There's an intimacy communicated through the body, being in presence together.

I was also struck by the last line because the dream ends with this very strong feeling of purpose: "becoming a translator is the best life path I can imagine pursuing." There's this affirmation, a sense of certainty and directionality.

Willow: As you say that to me, I'm aware of two truths at once. I do feel this sense of certainty, on the one hand, and I also feel this recognition of equality, on the other hand. This recognition that there's a fundamental ground of equality of all life paths, including the ones that I've been on thus far and the ones I might be on in the future. This sense that both truths led me to this point and that it is about being in communion with all beings' life paths. So those two truths arise as you point that out.

Eva: If this doesn't resonate, we can let it go, but it occurs to me that that sense of equality and also of multiplicity has occurred in other dreams we have focused on—the last one being the one about Eigen where you are both student and teacher (see the "Eigen Devi Dream" later in this chapter) and also the Jennifer One-as-silk dream about the professor in Marin (see Chapter 5). In apprenticing those dreams, I remember the feeling that whatever you choose to do you are enough as you are. They reminded me of that same feeling of wholeness in the dreamer.

Willow: Multiple aspects of the self, that they're all possible, that they're all integrated. That this way could be the path. And this other way could be the path and that there isn't competition between the parts.

That all parts can be accepted on the path. That none of them need to be left behind.

Eva: I recall the car image in the [Jennifer One-as-silk] dream: the car breaks down and you have to shift gears. Here there is also a vehicle. And I'm thinking of *vehicle* in the Buddhist sense: a system of beliefs and practices that lead you on a path of liberation from suffering. The vehicle needs to find its sustenance, to find its way.

Willow: Can you say more about your understanding of the vehicle in the Buddhist sense, to elaborate that association?

Eva: In Mahayana and Theravada, Buddhism is seen as a great vehicle. Through one vehicle, the aim is to become a Bodhisattva and help all sentient beings experience freedom from suffering. [Through] the other vehicle, the aim is to attain enlightenment, fully exiting the wheel of suffering.

Each form of practice is a vehicle through which transformation can happen.

Willow: What's coming up for me as you say that is the same idea—that all parts of the self can be welcomed on the path, that all three vehicles (Hinayana, Mahayana, and Vajrayana) can be welcomed on the path as well, that we don't have to pick and choose one over the other. All three vehicles can be welcomed at once—which goes to the heart of Rinpoche's teaching methods as I've practiced them. In the same way that all spiritual paths, across different secular and faith traditions, can be welcomed.

Eva: Yes, there may not be a hierarchy of vehicles.

In this dream, you encounter people from college (Jamie and Tim), an earlier time in your development. You are trying to figure out what vehicle will support you in moving through life. Where will this vehicle carry you, at that seminal age of trying to find direction?

I'm curious if the exam felt conditional, like if you didn't pass it, you would lose a certain respect or relationship?

Willow: I feel this sense of one-pointedness. Like, it's essential to listen, practice, respond, in the moment, and trust, have faith, in all that has been taught. And take a leap that my original expression will serve the moment.

And I think of Buddhist master Tsongkhapa's expression that "this life is like the tiniest drop of a rainbow, disappearing even as it comes into being." That feels like the right relationship to the oral exam.

Eva: Beautiful. Could you tell us who Sarah and Mary are?

Willow: Sarah, I associate with the Bible, although I don't consciously know much about her. I know she was Abraham's wife in the Hebrew Bible or Old Testament. I would be curious to learn more about her, how she figures in the Bible. And Mary I associate to the doubleness of Mary: the mother of Jesus and Mary Magdalene.

Eva: These female archetypes bring in another dimension of religion and faith. Perhaps another form of translation.

Willow: Thank you for that.

Eva: The choreography feels intentional. What else is calling you? What else feels like it has residue?

Willow: I guess I would just add that what strikes me in the dream is Rinpoche's multilingual capacity. That he's able to move from Tibetan to English, and that in the world his teachings are translated into many languages through his mandala, the Marpa Foundation. It feels quite meaningful to note that. There's direct communication that expresses itself across many languages.

Eva: You are so inspired that the conclusion of the dream is that you can't imagine a better path for yourself than becoming a translator. Such a beautiful dream. What else do you wish to speak to?

Willow: Just gratitude for my being able to share it with you here and receive your questions and to be able to do this work of transcribing and sharing the dream in our dream book.

Eva: Yes, it makes me realize that the process of translation is such a fragile one, to translate a night dream into the waking realm. I think it can be vulnerable—that translation process—because a dream can feel so emotional and so vivid and alive … who's to say it did or didn't happen. It is real in its own phenomenological way. I think the translation process can be delicate in terms of what we choose to communicate or not communicate with someone beyond ourselves.

Willow: Yes, I feel that delicateness in offering this dream through our book to the reader.

Dream Translation

I have longed for a way to express my gratitude to Khenpo Rinpoche for receiving me as a student and offering his blessings on the path.

The grace of this dream is to more consciously consider my teaching of psychoanalytic psychotherapy, integral relational psychotherapy, and transpersonal psychotherapy, as dimensions of the nondual un/conscious, to graduate students at the California Institute of Integral Studies and elsewhere, as a vehicle for passing on my study of Rinpoche's teaching—albeit in a translation from Buddhism to psychotherapy issuing from an omnist[19] regard for the common and distinct wisdom that flows from each spiritual tradition.

The presence in the dream of Buddhist, Jewish, and Christian mystics, in the dream figures of Rinpoche, Sarah, and Mary, is a welcome and healing constellation, helping me to ally the Buddhist, Christian, and Jewish streams of teaching influence in my life and in the world. *Sarah and Mary arrive at the door to help me translate. Rinpoche retreats, yet I introduce them to Rinpoche, who talks to them in English.* In these ways, there is dream collaboration and support among the spiritual lineages.

Receiving the medicine of this dream, it feels like a message of acknowledgment and permission and even encouragement to link, connect, and engage among these mystics of multiple lineages, for the benefit of their combined wisdom in the world through translation work. This brings me a sense of peace where I have felt conflict.

Also, from the perspective of nested dreams, it is quite meaningful to recognize that my study with Ken Wilber was a doorway to study with Lama Palden Drolma, which was a doorway to study with Khenpo Rinpoche. And the great difficulties I experienced with integrating the fruits of my study with each of these teachers delivered me to study with psychoanalysts James Grotstein and Michael Eigen. So the elliptical circle of genuine learning from dreaming continues to open …

Dreaming Lama Palden Drolma

Eva: My teacher, psychotherapist, and soul activist Francis Weller speaks of apprenticing sorrow[20] as a way of deepening our relationship to the soulfulness of the world. Grief is not simply an emotion, but an initiatory experience that can bring us into deeper embodiment and aliveness. By companioning sorrow and intimately learning from it, we can open more fully to all of life, this radical experience of being human, in a living-breathing interconnected world. Our relationship to grief strengthens our capacity to be with heartbreak and the inevitable losses and pain of being human as much as it evolves our capacity to open to joy, awe, and beauty. Mainstream culture tends to be phobic toward sorrow, but in avoiding it, we shut ourselves off from the ways sorrow can break open our hearts and ultimately transform us into elders able to be stretched large by grief and praise. In apprenticing sorrow, we become students of wisdom.

Willow: What you just said about apprenticing sorrow is a good place to start before reading the dream. Your expression clarifies that our work is about apprenticing Grace, apprenticing the dream, in order to be a student of Grace, to be a student of the dream, and to learn from the ongoing emergence of the dream. What you just said about apprenticing sorrow, which you learned from your teacher, Francis Weller, is a key ingredient of apprenticing Grace. And apprenticing sorrow is a key property of learning from nondual love. Nondual love is about apprenticing sorrow as well as joy; apprenticing sorrow is an instrumental part of apprenticing Grace.

Eva: Yes, sorrow is absolutely included.

Willow: So this is a dream entitled "Dreaming Lama Palden Drolma," or "Palden" as she's affectionately called.

There's an opening reflection to the dream that I wrote: *"Our dreams are closer than our eyes. They are sustained and revealed in love. This is why sometimes we cannot see them."*

This is the dream:

> *Dreaming that I connect with Palden in our classroom, I ask, with students present, when did Sukhasiddhi*[21] *open? I have not prepared for the class, and I listen to my intuition. We go to confer in the office. I realize Sukkhasiddhi opened just a few years before I joined. She [Palden inseparable from Sukhasiddhi] says she is sorry I wasn't there for the January birthday celebration. I say I was there. It is healing to be reunited and begin teaching together.*

Eva: Thank you. As you recall the dream, what are the latent feelings that carry over from the original dreaming of it?

Willow: One feeling is definitely sorrow. I've been away from the Sukhasiddhi Foundation, where I started as a student in 2006, for some time. And this dream is very healing because it provides a reconnection to my teacher, my Lama, and the stream of teachings that flow from Sukhasiddhi and Niguma. So there's definitely an apprenticeship to sorrow that comes up as I speak the dream, in terms of separation, loss, and reunion.

Eva: And is Lama Palden alive now or is she an ancestor?

Willow: She teaches presently, at Sukhasiddhi Foundation, in Novato, California.

Eva: So there's not only a union or a yoking of sorrow and grief at the separation, but also a joy at reunion as well. That's interesting because it's in tandem, a separation and a reunion at the same time in the dream—feeling the separateness and feeling the togetherness and the reconvening.

Willow: Yes.

Eva: I was also really struck by the fact that you taught from your intuition. That feels like a theme that also carries over from the Jennifer One-as-silk dream, dropping into the sense that you are enough and you have what you need already within you at this moment. You don't need to go off and do a bunch of research before teaching. And I wonder whether that's part of Lama Palden's transmission to you, to trust in your own intuition?

Willow: Yes, I'm keenly aware that *Lama* means spiritual mother.

Eva: Beautiful.

Willow: And … I am thinking of the Dalai Lama. *Lama* can be translated as the mother of all Buddhas.

Eva: Beautiful.

Willow: And *Lama* also means true liberation—genuine awakening from the heart of the Buddha.

Eva: I'm appreciating that Lama is used across genders in the Tibetan tradition, but I wasn't aware that it signified mother, that maternal nurturing instinct.

Willow: Yes, I think that's an important point—that it's a term used for all genders. I am reminded of the Buddhist teaching that all beings have been our mothers in the past.

Eva: The teaching is to have reverence for every being. Even if it's not a human because it could have been our mother.

Willow: Yes—the teaching holds true for all beings, for nature, animals, and humans.

Eva: I'm reminded of a scene from the Korean Buddhist film, *Spring, Summer, Fall, Winter… and Spring*. It's a really exquisite and meditative film. There's a scene where the Buddhist master instructs his student, a little boy, who is mistreating a frog. And the master provides that teaching—that the frog could have been an important ancestor that has returned in this particular reincarnation. It's a really tender scene where the little boy's consciousness shifts.

Willow: As you associate to movies, it makes me think of the movie about the Dalai Lama called *Kundun*.

Eva: As a student at Stanford, I helped curate a Buddhist film festival. Both of these films were included, but I haven't seen either of them for half a lifetime. I recall both being very powerful transmissions.

Willow: I'm aware of Thomas Ogden's paper (2016) on talking as dreaming, in the psychoanalytic literature, as we're speaking.

Eva: Oh, say more, since I haven't read it.

Willow: He just offers the teaching that talking is a kind of dreaming.

Eva: Because through talking, we freely associate. It's kind of a dance between, in this case, two entities. Most of life is just flowing forth without script.

Willow: Yes. I think about my colleague Steven Bloch from South Africa and his paper entitled, "Music as Dreaming: Welcoming Absence through Music." The paper (Bloch, 2024) centers on how music performs the psychological work of simultaneously figuring and symbolizing, working through, and nakedly presenting absence.

Eva: Intriguing.

Willow: The figuring of apprenticing sorrow as an inextricable dimension of apprenticing Grace, apprenticing dreams, feels quite important in terms of learning from nondual love. That apprenticeship is about letting go and about continuity—at the same time. About letting go of the appearance of a particular form of the dream while simultaneously being instructed by it.

Eva: Maybe it's just the phase of life that I am living through, but I've certainly been noticing that a large percentage of the dreams that live through me, in the night particularly, could be categorized as grief dreams. I sense that grief that is harder to metabolize in the daytime is worked through in the dream realm. It's an opportunity to reencounter a person in a slower, deeper way.

Willow: I'm aware that dear friend, psychologist, and artist Vipassana Esbjorn-Hargens[22] (personal communication, 2022) is doing research on people's experience of receiving messages from their departed loved ones. And I'm aware of how that happens in dreams. I'm thinking about memories as dreaming, as a kind of thinking—remembrance as a particular form of dreaming.

Eva: It occurs to me that the people who appear in our dreams may have passed, and some of them are still living, yet not occupying our daily lives anymore. And in that sense, there can also be grief. There's some loss there, whether it's a friendship or a teacher, an ancestor, a lover.

Willow: A pet.

Eva: Yes. Absolutely.

Willow: And this is the core of awakened heart that the Dalai Lama teaches about as Bodhicitta.

Eva: Do you want to say more about that for people who may not know what that means?

Willow: *Bodhicitta* means awakened heart. I think it's about honoring the heart of sadness that links us to all beings. By going into the heart of sadness, of suffering, we are yoked to one another. We're linked; in this way, we're never separated.

Eva: It is often our sorrows and losses that have us feeling the most isolated and the most separate. It feels so deeply personal. But what you're saying is that our sorrows and losses are actually what universally connects us in living through this fragile, delicate, beautiful, and harrowing life—that we all endure losses, including the loss ultimately of our self.

Willow: The body.

Eva: Yes, the body. And Francis Weller, who you referenced before, my teacher—apprenticing sorrow was his phrase—he also talks about apprenticing your own disappearance.

Willow: Can you say more about that?

Eva: I can speak to it in terms of how I understand it. I think it's living with this recognition that our time here is so temporal, so impermanent. It's about not getting attached to our egoic selves and being the masters of our lives. That actually we hold within us the knowledge that we are going to someday disintegrate and become part of this greater mystery, part of the cosmos, that we're never separate from it. We inhabit our bodies, our lives, and our relationships with the awareness of our temporality, which in turn, deepens our presence.

And I think that also relates to nondual love as I understand it because we're not seeing ourselves as separate from life or death. We unfold back into all of it. And also the capacity to feel joy as well as the capacity to feel sorrow and grief, that it's not one or the other. There's not a duality there. To be able to feel great joy arises out of our willingness to experience great sorrow. And I think it works the other way around too. We're not cutting ourselves off to any dimension of the heart.

Willow: That's beautiful. Thank you.

Eva: There was one question I had actually.

Willow: Yes?

Eva: About Lama Palden saying, "I didn't see you at the birthday celebration." And then you said, "I was there." I was curious how you understand that.

Willow: That's a great question. There's something about Tara's presence, which is Lama Palden's name. Her name *Palden Drolma* means *Tara*, which is the Savioress, the mother of all Buddhas. And she says, "I didn't see you." And I say, "I was there." It is about being both seen and unseen.

Eva: Like each of you becoming teachers to each other?

Willow: Yes. For me, part of the teaching of grace in this dream is exactly what you're pointing out. That the blessing that happens between teacher and student is always a mutual blessing. That the teaching of nonduality is exactly as you say, it's mutual.

Eva: I've certainly found that in the therapies in which I've been in the role of therapist. There comes a point when the work deepens and the relationship feels very mutual. Both participants are learning from one another. There's that recognition of, "Oh, look what we're discovering together."

Oftentimes I feel like that's when the client is, to me, being the carrier of wisdom. This happened recently in a session where we've been working together several years, and it occurred to me, "Oh, no, there's not a duality at this moment." We've arrived here because it's been a mutual exploration, and I've been as changed by it and surprised by it as the client has been.

I feel like the duality of somehow me being further along the path or being in the teacher role is just an appearance. In actuality, we arrive at the same juncture; we're walking the path with the same coordinates. And then it shifts again in different directions. But I've often found that's really when I feel most grateful for the work of therapy, when the duality dissolves.

Willow: That disappearance or dissolution that you spoke of.

Eva: Yes, where both participants are just feeling into this very mysterious human experience. And arriving in that moment of recognizing how fragile and radical and unusual it is that we're just two people trying to understand things that may be unresolvable. So those are the moments that make it all worthwhile, really. And those are moments of grace.

Willow: What you're speaking of is an offering back to the unborn, undying.

Eva: Something eternal? Yes.

Willow: Something that is ungraspable.

Eva: I've been in conversation with a friend who's been searching for a therapist for quite some time and feeling like she's met with a number of therapists who she feels either try to bypass her grief and have her focus on things that are positive or are trying to come up with solutions too prematurely. And it occurs to me that I don't think there is a lot of training for therapists to really just dwell in the space of the unknown.

I would say probably most therapists don't get that training.[23] I could be wrong.

Willow: I think you're quite right about that.

Eva: I've been feeling with her, the sense that people just want to fix her. And we talked about the sense that maybe they're not really comfortable sitting with her grief, or they don't really want to go into the depths. They want to stay in the shallows because it's too uncomfortable. So I think it's a certain art form actually, of being able to travel into the places where things aren't very clear and yet not needing to resolve it quickly for a person.

Willow: For me, this touches on the awareness of background presence, or background support—what James Grotstein (2000) wrote about in his chapter on the "Ineffable Nature of the Dreamer," from his book *Who Is the Dreamer Who Dreams the Dream*? He wrote about the importance of companioning background presence in therapy. It was Ofra Eshel who pointed out to me that we, as the therapist, are the conduit for that background presence (personal communication, January 4, 2024). So part of our job is to contact that background presence in our own experience. In just the way that you touched in with your teacher, Francis Weller.

Whoever it is that we have at our back in the consulting room, so that we're not alone in being a therapeutic ballast for others, that we are supported—that's who we contact. And I think that's a really important part of apprenticing Grace in therapy.

Eva: I definitely feel the lineage of certain soul teachers, certain supervisors, of course, and then also colleagues such as yourself, as holding us in an interconnected web.

Willow: I think calling them all in—supervisors, therapists, teachers, colleagues …

Eva: Lamas.

Willow: Back to that idea that all beings have been our mothers in the past, that all beings are Lamas, all beings are teachers.

Eva: Including our clients.

Willow: Yes.

Eva: I think about certain clients. Even in my dream last night, a client from the past appeared and I woke up this morning feeling that connection, but then also the loss that I can't just call up this person and say, "Did you have your baby? How are you doing? And how are things evolving?"

So I do find that dreamscapes are this place where you can not only meet again, but also acknowledge the loss and the change in the relationship. I guess that's why so many dreams do have that undertone of grief, as I think about it. Because there are often people that I'm not just going to call back up on the phone and say, "Oh, I had this dream and I was thinking of you." I recognize that contact actually stays in the dream. The encounter is meant for the dream realm. And there can be grief in that. And I don't know if that's part of your experience of re-meeting Lama Palden, meaning you're not going to call her up on the phone just now. The encounter stays in the dream.

Willow: There's a meaningful teaching in the dream about how there's no boundary in the dream.

Eva: Between student and teacher as you're coteaching? Yes. I imagine that is what Lama Palden would impart in you to carry forward.

Willow: Thank you.

Dreaming a Teacher and Their Teachings: Ken Wilber and the Integral Mandala

This is a dream in three parts. There's the nighttime dream; there's the afterward of the dream, which is the opening of the dream sequence; and there's waking from the dream. This is the third dream in this series about teachers and nondual love. And although it is the third of the four teaching dreams presented here, Ken Wilber was my first teacher among the four.

Here is the dreamscape …

Dreaming Upon Waking

Part One: In the Afterward of the Dream

In the same way that the khata (a Tibetan Buddhist scarf honoring a teacher, honoring Buddha nature) is white or multicolored, there is a diamond heart and a kaleidoscope heart. The clear and brilliant diamond heart of dreaming is none other than the self-liberated kaleidoscope heart of dreaming.

The more we become who we already are, the more we can give to others the gifts that we are here to create and to offer.

Part Two: Dreaming an Integral Mandala

On May 16, 2024, I dream that Ken Wilber has a younger brother who is also named Ken, and also a sister. His brother wants to join me. His sister is all right with that. His younger brother is a nightmare, in the sense that he won't quit. He has the ability to realize dreams on the spot, which is maddening. The sister observes that I know nothing about their father. The implication is that the father has been split off from the children out of a need to protect the children and that I had better respect this truth or be killed.

I can feel the dream's potency even as I am aware I have forgotten most of it upon waking.

Part Three: Upon Waking

> *Upon waking, in the morning, my husband Daniel brings me two imaginary friends, the ocean girl and the quiet girl. The ocean girl is the presence of the dreaming sea/see (as an aside, the* Dreaming Sea[24] *is also the title of one of my music albums). The quiet girl remains silent in order to hear everything—like a conch shell to the ear, hearing the sea's roar.*
>
> *It is a new day at home.*
>
> *We prepare to say goodbye to Sister Dolores, an Irish Catholic nun, a spiritual friend who has deeply supported our wedding, who is leaving the San Francisco Bay Area for Los Angeles. I see Our Lady of Guadalupe—a figurine that I bought to replace my Quan Yin/Kanzeon statue with—resting on my bedside table next to my alarm clock.*

Dreaming Integral Mandala

That's the montage of "in the afterward," "dreaming," and "upon waking." Each part of the nested dreamscape is like a poem linked to the whole. "In the afterward" begins with a description of the *khata*, which is the Tibetan Buddhist scarf that's offered to a teacher as a way of recognizing "perfect purity"—which is to say that it is this sense of recognizing the Buddha nature of the teacher that is also in the student.

There's rich symbolism in that doubleness of the khata's material reality (that it can be either white or multicolored), which I'm sure has been described by many for time immemorial. What I take away from that doubleness is that, on the one hand, there's the Buddha nature that recognizes that which transcends person, time, place, space, and in that sense is almost otherworldly. While, on the other hand, the multicolored khata, by signaling its inverse of all time, all people, all places, the fulfillment of all reaches of space as multicolored, feels like it demonstrates the Buddha nature of all existence and manifestation, of this world, of this earth. In my beholding those two symbols together, both the white otherworldly khata and multicolored earthbound khata, a more complete understanding of "perfect purity," of Buddha nature, comes into view.

In the afterward of the dream, regarding both the white and multicolored khatas, I liken those two aspects of God (Buddha nature, suchness, realization of any religious or nonreligious stripe) to the diamond heart and the kaleidoscope heart—the *diamond heart* being the quintessential symbol of Buddhism in many ways, and the *kaleidoscope heart*[25] being what I found in the secular world as a metaphor for this same divinity. Both hearts regard the perfect purity of all things, transcending and yet inclusive of and embracing all manifestations. I first discovered the album and song *Kaleidoscope Heart* in 2024, having presented at a conference at the California Institute of Integral Studies on the "kaleidoscope heart" in November 2023.

Willow: That's how I hold that sense of the afterwardness of the dream. I'm curious how it speaks to you?

Eva: First of all, I just want to say that I really appreciate how you're creating this nested dreamscape, or this montage as you say, and that the dream isn't this discrete phenomenon that has a beginning and an end and then we move on into "real" reality, so to speak. Because our dream life carries over and permeates and weaves throughout all aspects of our lives if we're conscious of it.

So many aspects of our experience—if we're open to that permeability upon waking and able to feel into that latent quality and energy in the dream—are touched by dreaming. That feels important to note.

Willow: I so appreciate you saying that—I feel like it's because of our collaboration that I'm able to thread these three movements of "the afterwardness," "the nighttime dream" itself, and "upon waking," and hold them together as nested dimensions of the ever-present dreamtime.

Eva: Yes. I was really struck by the phrase where you say that there's the "self-liberated kaleidoscope heart of dreaming."

In that sense, the dream itself has this wisdom that's inherent to it: the self-liberated kaleidoscope heart of dreaming. The more we become who we already are, the more we can give to others the gifts that we are here to create and to offer. The dream is a source of pure wisdom, the mirroring of those essential gifts.

Willow: The second part of the dreamscape, the nighttime dream, dreaming an integral mandala, is striking to me in the sense of presenting so many family relations: Ken as teacher, Ken as younger brother and sister, and talking about knowing nothing about the father, and splitting off from the children. There's a way in which the whole dream is like an ever-present family system, a family lineage.

Eva: When I hear *father*, I also think of it in a religious sense, father being the God figure.

Willow: Yes.

Eva: And that he's split off and unknowable. We don't know his face.

Willow: In many ways, this dreamscape and the nighttime dream within it point to my relationship to Teacher, with a capital *T*, in the archetypal sense. In my "real" life, I came to study with Ken in 1996. I studied and collaborated and worked with him through 2007–2008. And I continue to teach his work to my students and to draw from and engage with his integral teachings—in conversation with other models, other wisdom traditions, and other understandings—as I continue to further develop my own integral relational psychotherapy and perspectives.

Across that time, in the same way that the other teacher dreams in this chapter demonstrate a kind of movement or evolution of relationship to the Teacher as archetype, what you just named is illustrative of my earliest relationship to Teacher as archetype through Ken—seeing the teacher very much as other, very much as separate, very much as someone and something to be guided by, to learn from, to access that which was other than who I was, in order to grow or expand or develop who I was.

In some ways this dream reflects that early developmental relationship to *Teacher* and some of the movements of it, which makes sense given that, in the lineage of the four teachers presented in this chapter, Ken was my first teacher.

Eva: Interesting.

Willow: In a way, I was the youngest, developmentally speaking and chronologically speaking, in relationship to Ken, among all the teachers whom I dream about in this chapter.

Eva: I'm curious what you make of the dream further fragmenting him into multiple selves? There's the younger brother who has the same name, and then also the sister, and that younger brother is a nightmare.

Willow: Yes.

Eva: And he won't quit.

Willow: Yes.

Eva: These different facets of the siblings are broken down into three.

Willow: Yes. I feel like we could say that the initial Ken Wilber image in the dream is the idealization of Ken, and that the dream is cutting through that idealization and bringing forward all the other aspects too. From this vantage, there is the sense that reading a dream can be received as reading every character or every image in the dream as an aspect of self.

In this way, it's like a dream of cutting through the idealized Willow (as Ken) and showing Willow as a younger brother. Willow has a sister. Willow is a nightmare. Willow has a father that's split off from the children. And Willow as the father, Willow as the children …

I can read all of those dream images as aspects of myself. (Certainly, from an integral vantage, I can also read all of those dream images as conversations with Ken and as conversations with the integral mandala, but intuitively, selecting the perspective of the dream images as aspects of myself feels like the deepest portal, in the present moment, to emotional truth.)

Holding this dream in view, from this vantage, I reflect on my earliest journey of regarding the Teacher and receiving the teachings—whether it be the teachings of the integral mandala or the Buddhist mandala—and the way in which those two aspects (Teacher and teachings) are quite linked for me. And holding the dream in awareness is bringing to light, as the afterward of the dream illustrates, not only the idealized or white pure khata, but also the multicolored khata, the khata of all facets of being and personality and characteristics and qualities. In this sense the dreamscape reveals that the teachings aren't about going somewhere else, or becoming somebody else, but they're about illuminating what's already here, who's already here. A dream realization is that it isn't about trying to get somewhere, but it's about being here. Which, paradoxically and ironically, is a *developmental process* to come to.

Eva: I'm experiencing reverberations with the "Jennifer One-as-silk" dream in Chapter 5. I believe that khatas are often made of silk.

There's a pure silk, a oneness, but then there's also the breakdown. Breakdown happens in that dream. And there are different selves who are presented in the dream. One is really having an actual breakdown.

As I recall, there's this hereness of "there's nothing outside of you" that you're supposed to be attaining and developing. It's you, in presence, that is enough. Am I getting that right?

Willow: Absolutely.

Eva: There's a similar transmission in both of the dreams—both in dreaming the integral mandala and dreaming Jennifer One-as-silk.

Willow: Yes. I'm also struck by the last line that I wrote: "I can feel the dream's potency, even as I'm aware I have forgotten most of it upon waking."

There's a sense that what I was able to recall and remember and write down about the dream is the tiniest fragment of a larger dream. And what stays with me is the essence of the larger dream, through the bit that I was able to write down and recall.

There's a sense too that that fragmenting of the dream is an integral part of the self-liberated kaleidoscope quality of dreaming—that we don't actually have to remember and recall, in other words "come to consciousness" about our dreams in order for them to impact us and to teach us.

Eva: Yes, I think that's so helpful to hear because there is something so powerful in that liminal state between sleeping and awakening.

It can be so hard to hold the dream in mind. Even if I decide I'm going to go back in the afternoon to try to record the nighttime dream, the potency of the nighttime dream starts to fade. But the feeling of the dream being powerful, being transformational in some way, is often what stays with me, even if I can't recall the dream dialogue or the details.

Willow: Very much so. And then the "upon waking" …

Eva: Yes.

Willow: When Daniel brings me the ocean girl and the quiet girl and presents each of them, it's like being with the imaginal realm in waking space. It is how waking imagination is another portal to dreaming. Imagination in waking life is another kind of access to dreaming, dreaming when we are awake.

The ocean girl and the quiet girl are again a kind of pair and a kind of inversion of each other in the same way that the white khata and the multicolored khata are a kind of pair and a kind of inversion of each other. The ocean girl is the presence of the dreaming sea, and the quiet girl is utterly silent. She holds her ear like a conch shell to hear the sea's roar.

There's a sense of the ocean as being this vibrant, dynamic movement captured in the image of the ocean girl. The quiet girl is very interior and inward and introverted, but they are two aspects of being, and certainly these are two aspects of myself as a being.

I appreciate the parallel of those two aspects in the "upon waking" and how they echo, in some ways, the two aspects of the khata in the "afterward of the dream." I'm wondering what you hear there.

Eva: I am thinking about Brizo,[26] the archetypal ocean goddess of dreams from Greek mythology, which we spoke of a long time ago. She was an ocean girl in some respect, going back to the mythology of her diving deep …

Willow: Yes. Brizo.

Eva: That comes up for me, as it did when I read the dream. Ocean girl is the presence of the dreaming sea (*S-E-A*). and see (*S-E-E*). I immediately thought of Brizo as that ocean girl.

Willow: Yes, she's a goddess of dreams and a goddess of the sea, one and the same. We can definitely hear her as a presence.

Eva: It doesn't seem random, that it's an ocean … that it's a watery realm that she accesses.

Willow: The realm of emotions. The source of emotional truth. Then the other goddesses/archetypes that make an appearance in the dreamscape, and "upon waking," are Our Lady of Guadalupe and Quan Yin/Kanzeon.

I kept a Quan Yin/Kanzeon statue on my bedside table for many, many years. She is a Buddhist goddess. In partnering with Daniel, who is Catholic—a progressive Catholic who practices the dharma, not the dogma of the tradition—I then came to engage a relationship with Our Lady of Guadalupe.

I remember seeing this figurine of Our Lady of Guadalupe, or Mary, in Fairfax, California. I took her home with me. It felt very meaningful to place her, to place this figurine, on my bedside table.

I gifted the Quan Yin/Kanzeon statue to a dear friend and put Our Lady of Guadalupe in her place.

There's a way in which they occupy the same psychic space; quite literally, upon waking, that's the image of the feminine divine that I see on my bedside table. They are deeply related in that way.

Eva: Yes.

Willow: There's another doubleness.

Eva: I don't know very much about Catholicism and its saints and its iconography, but I would venture to guess that there's overlap with the Quan Yin/Kanzeon representation.

Willow: At root, I think of them both as being guides in the realm of compassion and faith and beneficence.

Eva: I suspected that would be the case. How is it for you to interchange these statues and form this relationship?

Willow: It's definitely a living practice—that interchange, as you say. It's very much about a kind of recognition of those qualities, of compassion, of faith, and of beneficence, and a kind of protection, a kind of guide to the sense of the other world or the other realms. I think of each of them, each expression of the feminine divine, as a kind of guide or threshold protector. I'm thinking of the late psychoanalyst James Grotstein who wrote *Who Is the Dreamer Who Dreams the Dream?* In his book, he talked about how every religion has its "threshold deities" or "threshold gods."

He used that word particularly: *threshold.* It really stands out for me in this moment that Our Lady of Guadalupe, or Mary, or Tara as she's sometimes called, are both goddesses of threshold crossing in that sense. They ferry one from one realm to another—of consciousness, of material reality, of psychic space.

And I'm also associating to your echo of the importance of a *threshold* or *doorway* in your listening to my dream of Khenpo Rinpoche …

There's a way in which having that interchange between Quan Yin/Kanzeon and Our Lady of Guadalupe/Mary teaches me about the links between those two traditions specifically, Buddhism and Catholicism, and also about the differences between those spiritual traditions and how they hold different icons and different expressions and stories and histories, and people relate to the two traditions from different cultural points of access and spaces. I think there's an embrace of *distinction-union* (as Michael Eigen authors the term) in that interchange between them.

Eva: I'm thinking back to the clear diamond heart—that there are different facets of the same gem.

Willow: Yes.

Eva: And all facets refract light slightly differently, but they're part of the same whole.

Willow: Yes.

Eva: Beautiful. Is there more that you want to share that stays with you, particularly from the heart of the sleeping dream, given that it's about your relationship to a formative early teacher?

Willow: I think about the aspect of the dream where it says Ken's brother wants to join me and his sister is all right with that. There's a sense of union with the Teacher archetype. Rather than what I first described as an early developmental sense of teacher as other, teacher as wisdom elder, teacher as guide whom one is learning from, there's something that this dream brings forward about joining, about union with the teacher in the sense of joining, in the literal sense of joining with the *guru* (the word the Eastern traditions would use for teacher, which is used particularly in the Tibetan Buddhist tradition that you and I have practiced).

This nighttime dream has all three of those aspects—teacher as other, teacher as self, and teacher as union. This recognition flows from the practice of *guru yoga*, a Tibetan Buddhist meditation practice where you see the teacher as everyone, everywhere, everything, and not as other than the Self/no-self.

Guru yoga is something that I practiced in the Tibetan Buddhist tradition as part of my studies of the lineage program with Sukhasiddhi and was expressed particularly in my studies with Khenpo Rinpoche. It applies here in the form of Ken as teacher too, in the sense of the Teacher archetype. The dream offers a way of regarding all teachers as vehicles of guru yoga, indivisible from self. All teachers as indivisible expressions of Self/no-self.

Eva: That makes sense. Even in the younger brother who is a nightmare, right? The nightmare as teacher too.

Willow: Yes. Exactly.

The dreamscape offers that it's not only the formal presentation of teachings, like in a classroom or a workshop or a seminar or a practice or a book, but it's also the interior communications of the teachings that you take from those methods of study and practice that actualize transmission. And the dream demonstrates that what your personhood and your personality and your own being does with all of that is radiant and churning and tumultuous and wonderful and terrible, all at the same time.

Eva: Thank you.

Willow: Is there any last thing that you might reflect about the dream montage before we close?

Eva: I want to go back to the dream words. I'm curious about the thread of respecting the truth about the father in his absence. And then the threat that you would be killed if you didn't respect that truth. I wonder what you make of that or … It was a very powerful word, to be killed off.

Willow: Yes. There is a teaching that exists in the world, and in Buddhism too, that in order to realize the teacher you have to kill the teacher.

Eva: Yes, that's right. "If you meet the Buddha on the road, kill the Buddha."

Willow: In order to recognize the teacher as none other than the wisdom mind or the guru mind of your own being, one has to dissolve two things—the teacher and the separate self. A student has to dissolve the sense of teacher as other, or we could say a student has to honor teacher as other that is distinct from the transmission of the teachings in a sense. You could look at it both ways: two truths. But I think ultimately, again, in the sense that all of the aspects of the dream and all the images in the dream can be seen as expressions of the self, it's really about killing the notion of a separate self.

It's like dissolving the sense of self as fixed, permanent, truly existent. Even as I say that, I appreciate in the doubleness of the white and multicolored khata, in the doubleness of the ocean and quiet girl, in the doubleness of Quan Yin and Mary, that there's this sense of "Yes. And …" There is a yes to killing the teacher and honoring the otherness of the teacher. There is yes to killing the notion of a separate self. And, from the perspective of the magic of illusion, there's a yes to honoring the separate self and so holding that doubleness.

Whereas I feel that from my experience with, or maybe from my limited understanding of the teachings of Tibetan Buddhism particularly, I feel like the apex of those teachings is often regarded as the cutting through of the illusory self. Whereas I feel, again, in my very limited understanding of Christianity as expressed in Catholicism, there is a core teaching about the sense of the self as child of God. As a unique self. And that there's an effort in the "upon waking" to hold both revelations (of the illusory self and the divine self) as two truths that are also interchangeable in a sense, refracting each other in a sense, contradicting each other from one perspective, but regarded as genuine illumination, as paradox, from another perspective.

Eva: Right, we wouldn't want to dissolve the self until there is a healthy self to dissolve. That could be really disorienting or even kind of maddening at a certain stage in development to kill off the self or say there is no self. At least that's my sense. We need to have a healthy self to then paradoxically see through the illusion of self.

Willow: Yes, taking that one note further, we need to recognize the God self, recognize the way in which the self is none other than an expression of divinity.

Eigen Devi Dream: Mystical Union and Partnering the Unknown

This is a dream from December 2, 2023, and I call it the "Eigen Devi Dream" in recognition of the two figures that stand out in the dream. One figure is psychoanalyst Michael Eigen, who has been a mentor of mine for the past decade at the time of this writing. I've been reading his books and I've been participating in the community of clinicians and laypeople who study and apply his work. I call that community a *mandala* to invoke the spiritual sense of a living field of deeply rooted interconnection. I've been a part of that mandala for the past decade plus. And in that context, I've contributed to scholarship on Eigen's work and its application through two volumes (see Fuchsman & Cohen, 2021; Daws & Cohen, 2024) and will be contributing to the forthcoming series on Eigen's work (see Daws & Cohen, 2026). In these ways, I've been actively engaged in Eigen's approach to clinical work and his thinking and its further applications.

The other figure in the dream is "Devi," which seems to come up only at the very end of the dream. And yet, I think it figures in the entire dream. *Devi* means goddess or a feminine spiritual being. And I think the dream, in many ways, weaves these two figures together because Eigen, for me, is not only a mentor and a teacher and a colleague, but also a being whom I regard as integrating the masculine and feminine spiritual capacities in psychospiritual work. And I often think of him at root as a "crazy wisdom" psychoanalyst, to invoke a Buddhist term for spiritual wisdom that has been used to describe Eigen. It is a multifaceted term that points to how confused mind and wise mind are both, in their true nature, none other than wisdom mind, however obscured or clear.

He figures in my own psyche, beyond all of these roles he inhabits, in two really interesting, complementary, and potentially conflicting ways. He holds the mantle of the masculine spiritual principle (which I would say is available to all people regardless of gender identity, expression, and embodiment), in that he is encyclopedic in his knowledge of psychological scholarship and academic prose and history and lineage.

I revere and admire that capacity and value his knowledge. Yet that kind of encyclopedic knowledge is not a capacity I bring to this world. And I hold myself as separate from that masculine capacity (which, again, I see as available to all people regardless of gender identity, expression, and embodiment) in some respects. Being true to myself and also being true to something I admire, it is humbling to acknowledge what my skills are and aren't.

And Eigen also holds the feminine spiritual principle in my eyes, in the sense that I feel that Eigen is deeply humble, even as he's also quite fearless in his outspokenness and leadership. In this way, I see the masculine and feminine capacities intertwined in Eigen, if we want to label complementary qualities of knowing and being in this gendered way.

And I regard him holding this deep feminine presence of psyche in that he really honors the emotional life of psyche and the depth of primal and primary process in a way that is unadorned, unscripted, doesn't have to be organized, can be wild and even chaotic and spontaneous and very awake and very direct. So I hold him in my psyche as holding up both the mantle of knowledge and the mantle of the spontaneous, unknown, unknowable psyche. And he weaves those two qualities in really beautiful ways that I have been magnetized to in my own teaching. So, I'm not surprised that I had a dream about Eigen and women and not knowing.

Here is the dream:

> *I am visited by a dream, about psychoanalyst and mentor Michael Eigen, of all the women in life that he knows and loves—culminating in love for his uncle, as a nephew, in the form of a musical theater production. The musical theater production is conducted as a lecture, during which, at first, the Stanford/NYU audience walks out on him, protesting his stance on valorizing "not knowing." But this happening paradoxically allows Eigen's circle of students to continue the production. Eigen swims in the university fountain and I jump in with him, in my black dress. The dream/Eigen teaches that every relationship has wounding and healing and every relationship implicates all other relationships.*
>
> *Dreaming that Eigen is old and young, fat and thin—multiplicitous—I sit "mistakenly" on the faculty side of the lecture hall. Then I claim a seat at the back. All my change spills out of my purse in coins. There appears a book that is on Devi.*

That's the whole dream, just as I wrote it from the dreamtime upon waking, staying true to exactly what was in the dream space. It first stands out for me that Eigen dreams of all the women in his life, culminating in his love for his uncle, as a nephew. So there's this play in transfiguration with gender. What next stands out to me is the form of a musical theater production as a lecture. So there's a play on art forms and pedagogy and pedagogical vehicles of musical theater production on the one hand and scholarly lecture on the other.

In "real life," Eigen teaches at New York University (NYU). And I was an undergraduate at Stanford University. So, not surprisingly, those academic communities meld in my imagination of an audience that walks out on his musical theater production, as a lecture, for Eigen's stance on valorizing not knowing. It's this part of me that feels terrified of being walked out on for not knowing.

But then, paradoxically, this walking out of the lecture hall allows his circle of students to continue the production. On the one hand, there is the production of clinical work, and writing about clinical work, that is happening through the vehicle of the Eigen mandala because of his embrace of not knowing. And in all of these ways, I can understand Eigen as standing in for a part of me as well as representing Michael Eigen the person.

I love that, in the dream, Eigen then swims in the university fountain. I'm reminded that there was a centrally located fountain on the Stanford campus that acapella groups would jump into as a ritual. I was a member of an acapella group called Everyday People[27] (we performed then, as the group continues to perform today, Motown, Rhythm & Blues, Soul, and other popular songs) while I was at Stanford, and I can remember jumping into the fountain. In the dream, I jump into the fountain in my black dress with Eigen. And I am reminded of the alchemical drawings and depictions of mystical union, the *coniunctio*, from the *Rosarium Philosophorum*, a sixteenth-century alchemical treatise, which Jung drew on to represent the alchemical process of therapy (Jung, 1966, CW 16). I feel like I'm touching the collective consciousness through this image of jumping into the fountain with Eigen. The literal image is of two figures, the king and queen, entwined in a stream; the dream image is like taking a bath in a fountain.

And then I'm really touched by this clear wisdom that the dream, that Eigen, teaches. Namely, that every relationship without exception has both wounding and healing,[28] and that every relationship without exception implicates all other relationships. That felt, to me, when I woke up, like the essential wisdom of the dream. I felt like "Oh, that's something very helpful to recognize, that part of me wouldn't recognize if not for the dream communicating that wisdom really clearly." That wisdom feels like something to contemplate, to ponder further; it feels like a deep emotional truth.

And then I appreciate this part of the dream where Eigen, or myself, where being human, we are multiplicitous. We are more than what meets the eye. We are not just young. We are not just old. We are not just fat. We are not just thin. We are all shapes, all ages. We shapeshift.

Then this last part of the dream I *could* read as a low-self-esteem dream image. I *mistakenly* sit on the faculty side of the lecture hall, yet in actuality, in waking life, I am currently a faculty member at the California Institute of Integral Studies, and I have been a member of three other university faculties in the past. But I think there's something playful about reading the dream as being about not taking sides. Like it was a mistake to take a side. And so I claim a seat at the back. Again, I could read it as a low-self-esteem dream, like I'm just hiding in the back. But I think there's something more significant about this phrasing: "I claim a seat at the back." I'm claiming the fact that I'm looking from the backseat and that feels advantageous. And it reminds me of the story of the Buddhas that lead from the front, Buddhas that lead from the middle, and Buddhas that lead from behind in the ship of life. There's something there about connecting with the Buddhahood of leading from behind.

And then there is this last line: "all my change spills out of my purse." All of my psychic changes literally spill out of what I might contain in coins, which is both a sense of treasure on the one hand, but on the other, also this sense of meagerness. Something not valuable and something valuable at the same time. It could be just a few coins. It wasn't silver dollars. But they were coins. They were a treasure.

The whole dream leads up to a book on Devi. The whole dream could be a commentary on honoring the multiplicitous psyche that doesn't know and yet knows directly. That is written in the voice of a feminine spiritual being. And I related, when I woke up, to writing this book with Eva and thinking about the grace of dreaming as a vehicle of Devi, which we both partner: awakened/awakening feminine spirit.

Dream Dialogue

Eva: Wow. There's so much richness flowing over from this dream. I'm curious, given that it's been a little bit over a month since the dream lived through you, what residue remains?

Willow: It feels just as alive narrating it at this present moment as it did when I dreamt it and woke up from it.

Eva: I felt that as you went through it. It's not like you've forgotten what certain parts meant or dismissed any parts. It all felt equally salient and potent.

My favorite line, which was so poetic in metaphor and image, "All my change spilled out of my purse in coins," because you could have written, "A lot of quarters or dimes fell out of my bag," but it was "All my change." The doubleness of, as you said, psychic change and transformation created this rich metaphor.

Willow: As you say that, it occurs to me that I can also view the Stanford/NYU audience that walks out as a part of me too, the part of me that walks out on the difficulty of not knowing.

Eva: As I listen to you share the dream, I couldn't help but see the dream as a trajectory of your own path from being an academic student at Stanford and through the Wright Institute and all of your academic training in psychology and how the introduction of Eigen's work, by his example and his mentorship, brought in a new paradigm for you of being with the unknown. This being with the unknown is in such contrast to being in the world of academia, which is all about building up knowledge and information and being in a paradigm that is securely planted in knowledge. Eigen introduced this other way of being and existing.

There's this playfulness between the lecture in the form of a musical and the spontaneous playful dive into the fountain. And so, it really feels like this integration of these parts of yourself between the academic who is firmly rooted in that tradition, and also the part who is able to really sit with the unknown and to appreciate the mystery. And that also feels represented by being in the faculty side of the auditorium and then the student side—that you are a perpetual student open to not knowing, open to learning, and that you value being both teacher and student.

And then, of course, psyche's incredible metaphor of all of your change spilling out of your purse. Change being both psychic, inner transformation, and of course the change of quarters and nickels and dimes. But this feeling of wealth—that you have access to both your academic side and your Eigen side, shall we say—it brings you a great deal of wealth that is overflowing from your purse.

And the other piece of this is also your approach to our book, originally being one that would be an academic book on dreams and the transformation you underwent to let that go and actually come into your own feminine wisdom, producing a book that is on Devi. So it feels like this dream also tells that story of the process that you've been engaging in.

Lastly, what does it feel like to be a woman that Eigen knows and loves? Eigen dreams of all the women in life that he knows and loves, so this definitely includes you.

Dreaming Devi

There is something alchemical in welcoming Devi according to the love of the masculine, from the inside and from the outside. My reverence for the masculine that partners rather than dominates, internally and externally in relationship to self and other, opens space to welcome the divine feminine.

Receiving the love of the masculine, within me and outside of me, is a transformative element of this coniunctio, or mystical union.

Since receiving this dream, I have opened to the presence of the divine feminine in a myriad of ways, known and unknown.

One of the ways this opening to Devi has figured is in our apprenticeship to dreams, an apprenticeship to Grace. I now recognize that to be an apprentice to one's dreams is to be a student of one's dreams, to learn from one's dreams. Not to master a dream, or to limit a dream's potential messages, or to imagine a dream could ever be fully interpreted or decoded. But rather to appreciate that *we live in nested dreams*—dreams within dreams within dreams into infinity. Akin to Stephen Aizenstat's (2006, 2011) work on dream tending, we do not seek to "interpret" the dream, or to "figure it out," or decode it. We seek to companion it, be in relationship to it. We seek to learn from the dream, not conquer it.

The dream, as psychoanalyst James Grotstein would say, is endlessly encrypted even as we realize some dimensions of it. Welcoming Devi, there is a deeper humility and a deeper reverence for the sacred that dreams usher.

In apprenticing dreams, we regard the transcendence of time and culture, while beholding and honoring the mystery of time and culture. As my friend and colleague Dr. Shalini Masih says, "Dreaming does not know differences … in geographical boundaries or in time" (personal communication, May 19, 2024). In this way, dreams are cosmic teachers and travelers.

We can apprentice our dream life as a direct, unmeditated spiritual teacher.

To apprentice a dream, we offer the dream to the circle—two or more present to receive the dream.

We practice awakening *to* the dream, not only from it, by apprenticing the dream, which is a feminine spiritual practice for all.

Here, we relate to the dream as a continuous awareness and mode of relationality, throughout the day and night.

Listening to your "hearing heart" (Eshel, 2019), notice what associations, links, connections, and related images that you hear.

As a guide to apprenticing the dream (Pearson, 2014):

See into and through the dream
Sing the dream that wakes you up
Rest in and as the dream

Dispelling and Living Dreams

Upon reflecting on these four dreams of four of my principal teachers,[29] nested within each other as they are, I have variously experienced my root spiritual teachers as dreams and as nightmares, according to the changing and dynamic dispositions of my own mind.

Dreams of longing. Nightmares of grasping. The path of devotion, true to the doubleness it can engender through the longings and yearnings of ardent desire, has taught me the wisdom of gurus as dreams that I have been inspired by and the delusion of gurus as ghosts that I have been haunted by.[30] Through the gradual opening into nondual love, where attachment gives way to gratitude and expectation gives way to appreciation, I have come to recognize and internalize the fountain of blessings that each of my teachers has graced me with, whereupon I can now stand proudly in the lineage of their teaching streams. I can offer the fruits of their teachings according to my own unique voice and understanding and my own spiritual authority and limitations, as I teach others in my roles as professor, artist, singer, writer, psychologist, and psychotherapist. For the dream of Self/no-self to release the mind of a hungry ghost and be enough just as I am, ever evolving, is a true grace. The difference of realizing nondual love has been a movement from seeking defined by grasping for attainment of knowledge to curiosity and discovery defined by wonderment that continues to open. For this revelation of nondual love, as ground and goal, I have each of my root teachers, and all of my teachers in this life (see Acknowledgments) to thank.

In welcoming the creative union of all my teachers and their luminous lineages, in an embrace of nondual love, dreams have become profound spiritual friends that recognize and reveal our true nature, in their casting, in their dispelling, and in their living.

From the perspective of psychoanalysis, dreams, as Freud said, are a "royal road to the unconscious."

From the perspective of indigenous wisdom, flowing from my Métis Cree ancestry, dreams are a conduit of Great Spirit in its myriad voices, guises, and expressions.

From the perspective of Buddhism, as taught by my Vajrayana teachers, meditating on the dreamlike nature of appearances, sounds, and thoughts is "illusion-like samadhi" dancing as emptiness opening.

From the perspective of my direct experience, flowing from realization born of mixing and combining these living meditations, dreams are, as psychoanalyst Wilfred Bion observed, a conduit of emotional truth.

Waking up *to* a dream of this life (including and transcending waking up *from* a dream of this life) is a supreme method of nondual love to which we are all continuously invited.

Notes

1 Visit https://www.naropa.edu/programs/graduate-academics/clinical-mental-health-counseling/transpersonal-contemplative-art-based-counseling/
2 Visit https://www.naropa.edu/profile/dale-asrael/
3 Visit https://integrallife.com/who-is-ken-wilber/
4 Visit https://lamapalden.org/about/
5 Visit https://www.sukhasiddhi.org/
6 Visit https://www.ktgrinpoche.org/about/biography-dzogchen-ponlop-rinpoche
7 Visit https://www.ktgrinpoche.org/nunneries
8 Visit https://www.ktgrinpoche.org/marpa-network/marpa-foundation
9 Visit https://www.wisdomsun.org/
10 Visit https://dpr.info/biography/
11 Visit https://seattle.nalandabodhi.org/
12 Visit https://vimeo.com/167226982
13 Visit https://as.nyu.edu/faculty/michael-eigen.html
14 Visit https://robinbagai.com/
15 A concept first advanced by D. W. Winnicott and built upon by Eigen.
16 Through this dreaming of nondual love (Almaas, 2023a, 2023b), Eshel's (2016, 2019) "delving into the profound mystery of telepathy at the heart of clinical psychoanalysis" as uncanny communication is extended to student/teacher/mandala experience.
17 Sean Esbjörn-Hargens, a principal student of Ken Wilber's, carries forth the best of further metaintegral teachings through his inspired work on the Varieties of Nonduality.
18 Visit https://www.ktgrinpoche.org/about/biography-dzogchen-ponlop-rinpoche
19 An *omnist* is one who values and sources the truth to be found in each faith tradition.
20 See Weller (2015).
21 Sukhasiddhi is both the name of a Shangpa Kagyu Tibetan Buddhist mandala founded by Lama Palden, Sukhasiddhi Foundation (see https://www.sukhasiddhi.org/), and the name of a completely awakened woman of the Shangpa lineage of Tibetan Buddhism,

from which, together with the awakened yogini, Niguma, most of the practices of Sukhasiddhi Foundation flow.

22 Visit http://www.integralhumanbeing.com/

23 Both Naropa University (https://www.naropa.edu/), where Willow studied and taught, and the California Institute of Integral Studies (https://www.ciis.edu/academics/department-clinical-psychology), where Willow teaches, are unique schools in their contemplative integral approach to training psychotherapists. Both institutions are built on a holistic view of being and becoming that honors the relationship between knowing and not knowing, fostering a lifelong love of academic and experiential learning. Spiritual practice is poured into and flows from the foundation of both schools. And, of course, genuine spiritual practice joined with formal education anywhere can provide excellent training.

24 Visit https://www.lionessroars.org/music/dreamingsea to hear this album, written, produced, and recorded with Eric Ramstad as The Watermoons.

25 See Sara Bareilles's album *Kaleidoscope Heart* and the song by the same title at https://sarabmusic.com/music/. "*Kaleidoscope Heart* is the third studio album and second major label album by singer-songwriter Sara Bareilles, which was released on September 7, 2010. The album debuted at number one on the Billboard 200, selling 90,000 copies in its first week."

26 Visit https://greekgodsandgoddesses.net/goddesses/brizo/

27 Visit https://acappella.stanford.edu/everyday-people and https://linktr.ee/stanfordeverydaypeople to tune into the music lineage of Everyday People.

28 For remarkable teaching on this recognition that relationships are at once healing and wounding, by virtue of our capacity to be both welcoming and obstructive to one another, see Daws and Cohen's *Primary Process Impacts and Dreaming the Undreamable Object in the Work of Michael Eigen: Becoming the Welcoming Object* (2024) together with Cohen & Daws's companion volume *Toxic Nourishment and Damaged Bonds in the Work of Michael Eigen: Working with the Obstructive Object* (2024). As an invited contributor to the first volume (see Pearson Trimbach [2024b]), I have been immeasurably helped by Daws and Cohen's teachings on the doubleness of welcoming and obstructive objects, through their vision for and stewardship of these companion volumes. In particular, see J. L. Eaton's chapters on "Welcoming Suchness" (Daws & Cohen, 2024) and on "The Obstructive Object" (Cohen & Daws, 2024).

29 For a more complete list of Willow's principal teachers, see https://www.drwillowpearson.com/contact

30 "Gurus as Ghost" is my further association to Shalini Massih's writing on "Ghosts as Gurus," which she shared with me in the form of offering further reflections on her book *Psychoanalytic Conversations with States of Spirit Possession: Beauty in Brokenness* (personal communication, September 2, 2024). See my review of this exquisite book (Pearson Trimbach, 2024a).

References

Aizenstat, S. (2006). *Dream tending: Techniques for uncovering the hidden intelligence of your dreams* [Audiobook]. Sounds True.

Aizenstat, S. (2011). *Dream tending: Awakening to the healing power of dreams*. Spring Journal Books, Inc.

Almaas, A. H. (2023a). *Love unveiled: Discovering the essence of the awakened heart*. Shambhala.

Almaas, A. H. (2023b). *Nondual love: Awakening to the loving nature of reality*. Shambhala.

Bloch, S. (2024). Music as dreaming: Welcoming absence through music. In L. Daws & K. Cohen (Eds.), *Primary process impacts and dreaming the undreamable object in the work of Michael Eigen: Becoming the welcoming object*. Routledge.

Cohen, K., & Daws, L. (Eds.). (2024). *Toxic nourishment and damaged bonds in the work of Michael Eigen: Working with the obstructive object*. Routledge.

Daws, L., & Cohen, K. (Eds.). (2024). *Primary process impacts and dreaming the undreamable object in the work of Michael Eigen: Becoming the welcoming object*. Routledge.

Daws, L., & Cohen, K. (Eds.). (2026). *A basic rhythm: Rebirth in the work of Michael Eigen*. Routledge.

Eshel, O. (2016). In search of the absent analyst: Commentary on Janine de Payer's "uncanny communication. *Psychoanalytic Dialogues*, *26*(2), 185–197.

Eshel, O. (2019). Would clinical psychoanalysis shy away from delving further into the unknown? On the mystery of telepathic dreams. *International Journal of Psychoanalysis*, *100*(3), 608–610. https://doi.org/10.1080/00207578.2019.1590121

Fuchsman, K., & Cohen, K. S. (2021). *Healing, rebirth and the work of Michael Eigen: Collected essays on a pioneer in psychoanalysis*. Routledge.

Grotstein, J. (2000). Ineffable nature of the dreamer. In *Who is the dreamer who dreams the dream?* Routledge.

Jung, C. G. (1966). The psychology of the transference. In W. McGuire (Ed.), *The practice of psychotherapy* (Vol. 16). Princeton University Press.

Masih, S. (2021). Reading the works of Michael Eigen: Artist of the invisible. In K. Fuchsman & K. Cohen (Eds.), *Healing, rebirth, and the work of Michael Eigen: Collected essays on a pioneer in psychoanalysis* (pp. 65–77). Routledge.

Ogden, T. (2016). On talking-as-dreaming. In A. Reiner (Ed.), *Of things invisible to mortal sight: Celebrating the work of James Grotstein* (pp. 97–114). Karnac.

Pearson, W. (2014). Dreaming. *Journal of Integral Theory and Practice*, *9*(2), 162–168.

Pearson Trimbach, W. (2024a). Listening to psychoanalytic conversations with states of spirit possession [review of *psychoanalytic conversations with states of spirit possession: Beauty in brokenness*, by Shalini Masih]. *Fort Da: The Journal of the Northern California Society for Psychoanalytic Psychology*, *30*(2).

Pearson Trimbach, W. (2024b). "Welcoming dreams." In L. Daws & K. Cohen (Eds.), *Primary process impacts and dreaming the undreamable object in the work of Michael Eigen: Becoming the welcoming object*. Routledge.

Weller, F. (2015). *The wild edge of sorrow: Rituals of renewal and the sacred work of grief*. North Atlantic Books.

10

DEPARTURE

Learning from Goodbye

The first time I met my partner's father, Brad was on a curb outside a hospital building as a nurse pushed him out the door in a wheelchair. Brad was suffering from late-stage Parkinson's, the disease damaging his motor neurons, unraveling his mind and, most of all, his dignity. Due to a complex cocktail of medications, Brad was seized by hallucinations that landed him in psychiatric care. I will never forget that upon seeing me, Brad burst into tears. I knelt on the curb, holding his shaking hand as we gazed at each other with wonder, both of us now smiling with wet eyes. Our first meeting felt more like a reunion, filled with relief.

I had arrived in Florida, a few days prior, at the very end of Christmas Day, 2018, with the intention of meeting Adam's mother, Lora, who was in hospice care. After retrieving me from the airport, Adam and I fell asleep in a nondescript motel on the side of the highway, awakening the next morning to the news of his mother's passing in the night. We lay silently in the cool shadows of the anonymous hotel room, our embrace a life raft drifting in an unknown sea. This was six months into our nascent relationship.

Because death dances in a mysterious duet with time, I intuited that Lora and I should not wait until Christmas to connect. On the Winter Solstice, Adam, sitting next to his mother in hospice, put the phone on speaker. I, three thousand miles away, had one chance to introduce myself—and also say goodbye—to my future mother-in-law before her soul exited this world. Adam simply listened as his mother and I forged a bridge between hello and goodbye. I promised as his partner that I would take the best care of him after she was gone.

> "That means so much as a mother," she responded. "I wish I had known you sooner, that I could have known you …" her voice trailing off into soft tears.

DOI: 10.4324/9781003591863-11

"But I do feel I know you in some way, and I really believe we will be tied together … always …"

Through my own tears, now audible over the phone, I said, "I know and feel your love, too, because of how Adam loves me."

"I'll take this love inside my heart wherever I go next," she said. As light faded into shadow, the deep indigo sky closing in, she gave us her blessing.

That conversation remains one of the most beautiful and sorrowful waking dreams in my life. I hold Lora's (un)dying wisdom in my heart: "In the end," she imparted, "it all comes down to love and presence." This emotional truth exists at the center of my marriage with Adam, a rudder guiding our small ship, a compass pointing north, reminding us of what matters most. This waking dream influences my sleeping dreams: from time to time, I speak with Lora on the phone; she is far away, her voice kind, her face unseen.

I share this context for the waking dream of this chapter because I entered Adam's family at a time of profound loss and transformation. In a letter to me just a few months before his mother's passing, Adam wrote, in response to pictures of ancient ruins I sent him while traveling in Greece: "*To me, ancient ruins have become powerful teachers of impermanence. At its height, the people of those civilizations must have thought their great structures would last forever. My family situation has certainly brought this up for me lately.*"

Entering into the fall of a family's "great civilization," I approached interactions with extra gentleness and sensitivity. As Brad's medications were adjusted, he was in a state of physical immobility in addition to his emotional devastation at the loss of his wife. Although we had just met, I recall his trust, allowing me to lift a spoon to his lips to feed him. I sat with Brad and Adam in a circle, holding hands as we pulsed small currents of energy between us. Creatively circumventing the limitations of his disease, we found ways to connect with tenderness.

Waking Dream

When Adam leaves his father's hospice bed in early December, 2022, Brad is unable to lift his head or make eye contact. Adam says his final goodbyes, not intending to return.

Then, on a winter morning in early January, Adam speaks to a hospice worker who reports that Brad may have "hours to days to live." Something immediately shifts within Adam. He books a red-eye flight for that same night. He arrives in Florida at 8:30 am and goes straight to his father's bedside.

Before Adam leaves for the airport, I let him know that I have several passages I could read to his dad over the phone, if he thinks it is a good idea. I wake up to a message from Adam, saying it would be nice for his father to hear my voice. I dial his number, feeling into the fragility of this moment. Brad is noncommunicative, but I trust he can hear me and take in the sound and tone of my voice.

I tell Brad how proud I am to call him my father-in-law, "my father-in-love." I remind him that the first time we met we held hands and sent a squeeze in a circle from Adam to him to me, pulsing love between our bodies. I ask Adam, who is holding him, to squeeze his hand again so that he can feel my love through Adam, moving into his body.

I read him "Entering Death" and "For The Dying," two blessings by John O'Donohue.[1]

I recite "Into A Large Existence" by Rabindranath Tagore:[2]

Peace, my heart,
let the time for the parting be sweet.
Let it not be a death but completeness.
Let love melt into memory and pain into songs.
Let the flight through the sky end
in the folding of the wings over the nest.
Let the last touch of your hands
be gentle like the flower of the night.
Stand still,
O Beautiful End,
for a moment,
and say your last words in silence.
I bow to you and hold up my
lamp to light you on your way.

I repeat Jewish prayers from chaplaincy, allowing the blessings to wash over him. I pause and listen to the silence between phrases, which feels thick and full of presence.

I begin to deviate away from the formal words written by mystic poets and philosophers. I follow my intuition and begin to guide Brad on his departure:

Thank you for raising an incredible son, Brad.

You can let go, knowing that from here onward, I will take the best care of Adam.

All of the love you have given in this lifetime will continue to live on in the love that Adam and I share.

It will live through us and circulate out into the world, into our friendships, into our family. We will continue to express your inheritance of love so that it lives on forever.

May you feel ease in your body, Brad.

May you feel ease in your heart.

May you feel ease in your entire being, Brad.

Allow yourself to dissolve into Love.

Allow yourself to be held by Love.

May you be held by Love.

May you relax fully into Love.

Each blessing emerges, arises, descends like gentle waves in the ocean. I pause. Brad listens. He inhales. He exhales. Silence. He takes his last breath on this earth. His soul releases and departs from his body.

Dream Dialogue

Eva: Everyday people are departing from this life, just as new beings are entering. Ordinarily, we don't dwell on this magnitude as we go about what's next on our to-do list. Being with the dying process, time feels thick and tenuous. We are forced to slow down and companion with the unknown, moment to moment.

I never had the privilege of knowing Brad before Parkinson's took up residence in his body and radically altered his relationship to himself and the world. Biology can be so utterly cruel. And as humans, we are forced to dig deep within ourselves to exist with what we think we can't possibly bear. This is where, I believe, religion and spirituality—and creativity—come into play.

As Brad's condition declined, so did his capacity to communicate. I remember a professor in graduate school explaining neurogenerative diseases as though the patient is living inside a glass home. Over time, the windows become more opaque as though Vaseline has been smeared across the glass. The patient, in turn, is trapped by their own isolation.

When Brad used to phone us, his thought process was often hard to comprehend; I sensed his efforts to assert order over an internal experience that was eroding and crumbling. I was able to stay present with him in a way that may have been much harder had he been my own parent.

I was extremely relieved when Adam decided to book a red-eye flight to Florida. I wanted him to be by his father's side; I felt this was the right decision. I told Adam that if in the morning his dad was still alive, I would like to have the chance to talk with him on the phone. I gathered that night several passages, poems, blessings, and prayers that I wanted to read to Brad. The next morning, I felt a heaviness permeating the empty house and my heart. I took a deep breath and got the courage to call Adam. I could hear a little bit of Brad's breathing in the background. I knew that Adam was there holding him as well as his youngest sister.

I entered Adam's family as an outsider at a moment of crisis; I hope my presence was a source of stability and support. I began cycling through these different prayers and reading different lines over and over again. I felt like we were entering a liminal space together. I wasn't entirely sure how to conclude the experience. I knew it was likely a final goodbye, and there was no script for what to say. So, I intuitively kept repeating different lines of the prayers and blessings. At a certain point, in my own words, I began to guide Brad, offering him permission to let go. I honestly didn't think he was going to pass during the hour I was with him on the phone.

We entered a kind of waking dream together. *May you feel ease in your body, Brad. May you feel ease in your heart. May you feel ease in your entire being, Brad. Allow yourself to dissolve into love. Allow yourself to be held by love. May you relax fully into love.*

I repeated the last few lines multiple times to him. *Allow yourself to be held by love.* And then he took his final breath. As I couldn't see his consciousness leave him, my own breath left me for a moment when I understood what had happened. I felt stunned with awe—awe that Brad trusted my guidance. It was an incredibly powerful and humbling moment when I realized that my words, my voice, were the last voice, the last words that he heard as he left the earth.

Willow: What are you feeling as you trace your experience with Brad and Adam?

Eva: As I recount the waking dream, I feel how we were really in sacred territory together. Even now, it feels charged with power and wonder. His passing will always be a mystery. Was he able to will the moment of his departure? I'd like to think that we helped create the conditions of safety and love that allowed him to let go with grace. Had I known he was going to take his last breath when I got on the phone to be with him, that would have felt like too big of a responsibility. But entering into the unknown together, that was something I felt perfectly capable of. That Brad allowed me to guide him, that he surrendered fully, was such an immense parting gift. He allowed me to trust in my own medicine as a spiritual guide.

It felt extremely natural to offer these "pointing-out instructions." Due to my own experience with unresolved illness in my young adult life, I've spent many hours contemplating my own mortality, feeling into the depth of my vulnerability in this body, which I view as a very temporary home. I've apprenticed my own disappearance, as my teacher, Francis Weller, would say. I've practiced my own death countless times, especially when I've been in the depths of physical pain. To counter the darkness in that place, I've learned that the only medicine more powerful than fear is love. Love has to become stronger than fear. I imagine being held by Divine Love, dissolving into love. My own practice made it extremely natural for me to offer these instructions to Brad when the time came.

I'm so grateful to Brad that he trusted me enough to do the bravest thing he has ever done: to let go of life and trust that love would embrace him in the unknown. Even as I feel a heaviness in my heart, recounting the dream, I also feel a deep sense of gratitude to Brad that we could enter into this sacred experience together.

Although Brad was forty years older than me, some of our physical struggles, in terms of neurological symptoms, actually overlapped. I could relate to his vulnerability and understood that his body was no longer the best vessel for his soul anymore. His departure, though incredibly sad, also felt, for me, a form of ultimate liberation: he would finally be free from a body that was harming him more than helping him. So I wanted to create the most graceful and loving send-off for him that I could, whether it happened later that day or the following week. The gift was that we journeyed through the transition in that hour together.

Willow: I'm really appreciative that even in departure connection can deepen. That even in this worldly perception of endings, actual deepening can occur, is occurring. And that our perception of the end is just an illusion.

Eva: So true. Thank you, Willow, for noting that. The waking dream really felt like an *initiation*, which is also a word for *beginning*. Clearly, this was an initiation for Brad as he entered through death's door into a realm beyond this one. And it was an initiation for me in that I had never guided somebody through the transformation from life to death. So it was a beginning as much as it was also a leave-taking. And yes, we absolutely deepened our connection. I feel closer to Brad as a result and this closeness lives on.

Willow: I'm curious to ask, in what ways you link that experience to a dream?

Eva: It is very much a waking dream. As it was occurring, I was aware of the dream state: being in the unknown and trusting in its unfolding together. I knew I was facilitating something, but I also felt like something bigger and more mysterious was coming through. I was listening to a higher source and collaborating with it through my intuition. I was aware that Mystery was holding everyone present in a liminal experience. Being with the unknown can be an extraordinarily sacred experience, if we enter it with reverence.

Most of our lives, we live with the illusion that we are in control. Awakening to a living dream is a profound acknowledgment that we actually don't know what is coming next. Being in the presence of the sacred requires a deep kind of listening. Death unfolds according to Mystery. We aren't in charge.

Liminality asks us to be fully present for whatever needs to happen without any agenda.

Willow: I'm thinking, as you're speaking, about the dynamics of listening, waiting, opening, cutting through expectation—that there's also the dimension of enacting, creating, bringing into being that I think is an equal part of the dream. The word that I've used in my writing is *fathoming,* as a way to think about imagining that what seems unimaginable could even occur on one side. Fathoming is a way of dreaming, imagining that something could be, opening a space for the possible. And the other side of that opening is creating. I've talked about it in my writing as original artistry, dreaming as original artistry in the sense of collaborating, collaborating between the unknown in us and the unknown outside of us, meeting and co-creating, as we are now as we converse.

Eva: Absolutely. You're right. As much as there was a presencing and listening, there was also an offering. I chose to speak particular lines of poetry, and I delivered them in a particular way. I began to speak my own poetry, what was arising from my own soul, including my own wishes for him. So, yes, there was an engaged collaboration with Mystery. The fact that I could not see Brad felt significant, too, because I was really listening in a different dimension without any visual cues. I was truly in the dark.

Willow: The other metaphor for being with the unconscious, which I've used in my teaching, is seeing in the dark. The way that we get up in the middle of the night and everything's darkened and yet we're having to see in the dark to make our way into the world, even though everything is occluded. I love how you said meeting presencing with offering. That it feels like dreaming is the collaboration between presencing and offering—presencing as the bridge between receiving and offering.

Eva: The offering comes from the psyche and soul. We have to practice presencing so that we are awake enough to receive those offerings.

Willow: And how does that dream live in you now?

Eva: Such a beautiful question. The dream continues to be a gift. It affirmed an invisible medicine that I have been cultivating through these years of my own illness experience. Although I am not as active in my career in the outer world, I have, however, cultivated direct knowledge through life experience with profound vulnerability. I wasn't afraid to enter that unknown space between life and death with Brad. In our culture, death is not something that many people want to talk about or be near. Because I've had so much time to feel into my own fragility and mortality, I'm less afraid of that territory.

The dream helped me to claim my own medicine, the soul skills I've been cultivating the last six years. As Brad trusted me, I began to trust the medicine. I am forever grateful to Brad for this gift. Being in the mystery of death with him was immensely powerful. We ventured through the veil, and I feel very connected to him as a result.

Willow: You created an altar, sharing your experience and holding of Brad's crossing over as a place of worship in your home with Adam, as a place of being with his passing.

Eva: Yes. I think it's so important that we have rituals and artistry to honor these thresholds. Death is so medicalized in our society. Hospitals, in my experience, are not places of spirit or healing. Unless one is lucky enough to have a death doula present or chaplain or skilled hospice worker, death can be a clinical experience shrouded in a lot of fear. This waking dream taught me that death can be a beautiful, even a healing, experience. Grief and beauty don't have to be separate.

Adam has expressed to me that as much as his father struggled and suffered for the final years of his life as he battled Parkinson's, his departure was filled with grace. I feel at peace in my soul knowing that we could facilitate grace for him. That he could be held in the arms of his son and daughter and feel, I hope, surrounded by love as he let go. Adam said it was a very peaceful experience. I wish death could be a graceful passage for all sentient beings.

Living the Dream Onward

As a child, I quietly carried *preemptive grief*, the fear that those I loved would one day not be here. Closely attendant with this grief was a deeply ingrained fear of separation. Years later, in my early adulthood, a therapist named this feeling as *inherited grief*. This made total sense to me as the grief I carried always felt so much larger than myself. Although it was rarely spoken of in my family, the transgenerational transmission of trauma from the Holocaust resided at the center of my psyche. I feared the future loss of family members, yet the fear also felt of the past, a knowing in my bones that these tragic and violent separations had already happened.

In light of this, guiding Brad on his departure was extremely healing for me. Companioning death, rather than dreading it, allowed me, and all who were present, to enter the dying process as a profoundly sacred, and even beautiful, experience.

Death is the ultimate encounter with Mystery. It's natural for trepidation and fear to arise when we face fully into the unknown. And yet, when we soften ever so much and stop bracing against fear, compassion and grace have the chance to enshroud us as we feel into our mortal fragility. Just as fear accompanies us into the great unknown, so, too, can a sense of reverence.

As Willow noted in our dialogue, death is not simply the end of life. Death is also a beginning, an initiation into spirit. Through the process of dying, deepening can occur: my relationship to Brad—and Adam—deepened, Brad's relationship to life and to love deepened, as did our relationship to divinity and spirit. I learned that grief is a soulful expression of praise for this precious, heartbreaking, ephemeral existence. As Francis Weller writes, "My grief says that I dared to love, that I allowed another to enter the very core of my being and find a home in my heart. Grief is akin to praise; it is how the soul recounts the depth to which someone has touched our lives. To love is to accept the rites of grief" (Weller, 2015, p. 25).

Entering the threshold between life and death, we find ourselves on sacred ground. The clinical and medical aspects of dying often obscure or negate the potential of the sacred. We revere birth with wonder. What if we could approach death similarly?

Many world traditions see death as another form of (re)birth, entering the *bardo*—intermediate state between death and rebirth—the space where the spirit meets Original Source. How paradoxically enlivening it was to be awake, moment to moment, to the living dream that is dying.

Ultimately, it is hard to know who was serving who during the transition of Brad's departure. I was serving him as a spiritual guide. And yet, Brad's trust in me was a form of loving service as well. He gave me the parting gift to trust in my own medicine, the intuitive capacities I have to offer and heal this fragile world in my own small way. My soul stretched ever wider, the pain of loss coupling with deep, aching love for the very fact that we get to love at all. Like any powerful initiation, Brad and I were both irrevocably changed.

The waking dream of my conversation with Lora on her hospice bed influenced the waking dream of me guiding her husband in his departure four years later. In the end, Lora imparted, "It all comes down to love and presence." The experiential wisdom of both of these waking dreams, a confluence of deep sorrow and beauty, loss and connection, continue to weave through the waking dream of my marriage to their son, Adam.

An image arose, only a few days after Lora died: Adam and I found ourselves on an abandoned beach. The fog was so thick, we could not see a few feet in front of us—a poignant metaphor for what it feels like to live beyond the death of one's parent. We held hands as we entered the fog, the sun shining through, creating an atmosphere of pure white light. Little by little the sun eventually dissipated the fog, land revealing itself in patches. Now, walking the same path in life as a married couple, Adam and I continue to meet the unknown together, taking one step forward at a time, entering the Great Mystery with loving awareness.

Notes

1 "Entering Death" and "For the Dying" are from John O'Donohue's *To Bless The Space Between Us: A Book of Blessings* (2008, pp. 178–179, 180–182).
2 From *The Gardener* by Rabindranath Tagore (Macmillan and Co., Limited, 1913). https://en.wikisource.org/wiki/The_Gardener_(Tagore)

References

O'Donohue, J. (2008). *To bless the space between us: A book of blessings*. Doubleday.
Weller, F. (2015). *The wild edge of sorrow: Rituals of renewal and the sacred work of grief*. North Atlantic Books.

11

BURIAL

Learning from Death—Île-à-la-Crosse

In this chapter, we cross the threshold of being on the other side of life. Here, we experience a nighttime dream about "new Île-à-la-Crosse" and a transcultural practice of caring for the dead by invoking burial rituals of two tribes that are in conflict. In "real life," Île-à-la-Crosse is a place in present-day Saskatchewan, Canada. It is the geographic location of the marriage of my great, great, great, great-paternal-grandfather and grandmother.[1] The contemporary landscape of war, foremost among them war between Russia and Ukraine and war between Israel and Hamas, contextualizes this dreaming the collective cry of the world soul—a cry for understanding across and among cultural groups.

I've titled this dream, from September 6, 2023, "Burial: Learning from Death—Île-à-la-Crosse." The dream itself is relatively brief, but it also feels like one that's most germane to how I regard dreaming as the synchronous past, present, and future. It also felt synchronous to be meeting with Eva to share this dream, as we had been discussing political instability on the world stage.

At the same time, I feel like this dream speaks to a way in which I'm relating to the present moment, and then also how this present moment also implicates the future. Of all the dreams that we have recorded and dialogued about and written about for this book, this nighttime dream feels like the most "recessed" dream for me. It feels both deeply important in terms of its personal expression of Psyche, as it relates to my own individual history and ancestry, and also in the way that I am connected to the collective.

It also feels like the most shadowy or effervescent or mercurial dream I have recorded for the book; this nighttime dream is very hard to figure, hard to grasp. It feels like a dream that is, at once, extremely close to me and at the same time very deeply rooted in the collective. In just this way, the nighttime dream seems to arise at a meaningful distance from my "personal" Psyche, tapping a deeper

DOI: 10.4324/9781003591863-12

collective layer of emotional truth that also is inseparable from my personal expression of Psyche.

This Is the Dream...

> *Burying the dead in one tribe. Wrapping the corpses carefully in deerskin. Sprinkling them with cornmeal. Saying prayers for safe crossing.*
>
> *These ritual blessings held in mind as another tribe dresses the bodies in another tribe's blessings. Carrying the dead to the new Île-à-la-Crosse.*[2] *Saying prayers in a new tongue: That there be an absence of war. That there be peace for each soul. Ferrying the bodies to the same Great Spirit.*
>
> I think, as I wake, *this is the grace of dreaming.*
>
> "*Ke sakihitin awasis*" resounds in my heart ("I love you baby," in Cree).

I am listening for caesura's cry:[3] listening for the place where the soul is torn. I am listening for the medicine right within the poison: listening for healing potential in the echoes, in the resonances of the soul's cry, of the soul's tear, of the soul's wound.

Here caesura's cry is to return to her home with the Great Spirit, on Earth and beyond this life. To do so, the dead must pass through the rites of two tribes, each in their own customs and their own language. The soul's cry is to be recognized, to be heard, indeed, to be honored by each tribe in the continuity of ferrying home the dead, beyond customary tribal boundaries, where Earth meets sky. This continuity of the ferrying home—realized on Earth—is the medicine, traversing the lines of cultural and social separation.

Dream Dialogue

Willow: On one level, this dream speaks to me of my link to Cree ancestry and Metís-Cree ancestry. *Metís* means "half-blood," or "mixed race," which links me to my great, great, great, great-grandmother, Charlotte Small who was Metís-Cree (see Trimbach, 2022 for ways in which I dream Charlotte Small Thompson). She was married to my great, great, great, great-grandfather at Île-à-la-Crosse, which is in modern-day Saskatchewan, Canada.

At the urging of the dream, prompting me to learn more about the history of Île-à-la-Crosse in the afterwards, I discovered that the Cree name for Île-à-la-Crosse is *Sakitawak*. As the Metís of the region recognize, at the confluent levels of identity and spirit, "Sakitawak is Cree for where the rivers meet and is the enduring name of Île-à-la-Crosse, Saskatchewan."[4] Specifically, I learned that there are three rivers that converge at Lac Île-à-la-Crosse: the Churchill, the Beaver, and the Canoe. The region was originally a borderland area between the Cree and the Dene Peoples, and "it became a meeting place that promoted the cultural and socio-economic exchanges of the Cree, Dene, Scots, English, French, and Metís peoples" (Macdougall, 2010).[5]

On one significant level, dreaming Île-à-la-Crosse is about dreaming the physical place, as a geography of my connection to Canadian ancestry and, in this case, my Metís-Cree lineage. At the same time, on another significant level, recalling that Metís "means mixed race or cross breed in French,"[6] I would say that dreaming a *new* Île-à-la-Crosse is about dreaming an *enduring* spirit that continues to *originally combine* cultural/spiritual heritages. This ongoing confluence of where cultural/spiritual rivers of identity meet feels like the essential emotional truth of dreaming the *new* Île-à-la-Crosse, as a yet enduring geographic and symbolic Sakitawak that both includes and transcends location.

Given Île-à-la-Crosse was the place that my great, great, great, great-grandparents were married (so the marriage of a Metís-Cree woman to a colonial man of European heritage, in Canada), it marks the symbolic joining of two tribes—in the collective and also in my own ancestral lineage. I feel like the dream itself harbors the theme of two tribes recognizing the same soul's journey—with two sets of customs and two sets of blessings in different languages that connect—representing both how the soul is torn *and how the soul is mended.* The dream feels like—for me, as I wrote it, and again now, as I regard it presently—like the essence of simultaneously receiving the grace of dreaming and bestowing the grace of dreaming.

Eva: There's a really deep and beautiful transmission through this dream that projects, as you said, a new meaning as we hold it in this moment. It is meaningful that as we dialogue about the dream today, it is a month-and-a-half past the time that you dreamt it. The passage of time between first receiving the dream and this telling of the dream now illuminates new meanings for us. Within the transmission of this dream, there truly is medicine for these current times we are living in. I found myself becoming tearful as you read the beginning lines around the second tribe using or expressing and enacting some of the first tribe's rituals to bury their dead.

As we witness and learn of so many deaths happening right now between two tribes, what would it mean if each tribe took some of the other tribe's rituals to know that grief is a shared experience known by each? The religions, the traditions between these two tribes, may be different, but the source of grief and the source of spirit where these bodies are going to is the same. I was feeling into not only the pain of the division between the tribes, but also the potential of sharing in the ritual of grieving the other tribe's loss as one's own.

Willow: I've been wondering about this presence of caesura's cry ever since Ofra Eshel wrote that term in an article about Bion's work. She asked, at one point in the article, "Is this caesura's cry?"

That presence, that invocation, that recognition, that concept, that reality, absolutely dialed in my awareness, in such a lightning-rod way, to think about how, on the one hand, as it's expressed in the dream, there's the division of lines of cultural and social separation, but on the other, there is the traversing of the lines of cultural and social separation. There is the tearing. There is also the potential for mending. Further, there is a living confluence, a waterway of the soul's passage, where the tribes may meet.

That is the separation/union of these two tribes.[7] There's something I feel the dream communicates: It's not about resolving some unified ritual or language or blessing, but rather it's about wrapping the bodies in more than one blanket, about the expression of multiple blessings and multiple tongues and multiple rituals that see their essence in each other in the way that you just beautifully described, while also honoring their uniqueness.

Eva: Which is to hold very real differences at the cultural level, and yet, I think at the spiritual level, to recognize and contact origins of sameness.

Willow: Yes.

Eva: I wondered when you shared the dream, which had so much tenderness—almost as if *you* were wrapping the cloths over this body and sprinkling the cornmeal, whether these are rituals that you actually know of, or was it the dream that introduced you to them?

Willow: I honestly don't know how to answer that question. I don't have any direct guidance or learning or instruction or recitation of wrapping corpses in deer skin and sprinkling them with cornmeal. But in my dream, those were the rituals of caring for the dead, and they felt very sacred and precious.[8] I felt that was part of the receiving, the grace of dreaming.

The dreams taught me something about sacred ritual that I could experience in the dream. This is something that my dear friend and colleague Robin Bagai said about dreams in his Eigen seminar recently, "Dreams afford us an emotional experience that we may not have in our waking day."[9]

Eva: Beautiful. I felt that as you described the rituals. I could feel the engagement of those rituals in my own body—the intentionality, the anointing, the care. Now, that is part of you. You actually did experience it, as you said, in the dream. What I have found missing during periods of deep grieving is not having a collective ritual. I feel the lack of the collective ritual profoundly, and in a way, your dream offered you that experience so that it is part of you now.

Willow: Yes, definitely. That felt like the bestowing of the dream that I was able to receive within the dream.

Eva: Yes, the grace of the dream. It felt embodied as you wrote it, as you described it. Another phrase that stood out to me was "half-blood," the other and the self and the self and the other, since we are living through such divisive times of "us" versus "them." Something about that had me feeling an integration of "it's not an oppressor versus an oppressed." Both of those realities exist within us, and you come from a lineage where you've inherited both of these tribal traditions and ways of knowing, and they exist, they coexist, within you.

Willow: In the case of Charlotte Small, she had both Cree and Scottish ancestry. Her mother was Cree and her father was Scottish. I feel like those two themes, the theme of twinship and the theme of the other within, are meaningful themes in the series of dreams that we're exploring in our book. There's the twinship aspect of your *Surrender: Learning from Illness* dream in Chapter 6, and the twinship aspect of the *Jennifer One-as-silk* dream in Chapter 5. I consider the other in the self, the other recognized within the self, as aspects of each of those dreams also.

Eva: Absolutely. I'm glad we're homing in on certain themes that are alive in these conversations because one of the gifts of dreaming is this sort of de-identification with self as somehow being this bounded entity. There's something so movable and changeable and all these permutations too, right? Everything that we dream is an aspect of us. For instance, there are certain interpretations of the dream such as *you* are the body being wrapped in the deer skin and *you* are the person who's anointing the body.

In a way, it is all a creation of Psyche where there aren't really the same boundaries between other and self anymore. It's like these are all aspects of being that Psyche is speaking, and we get to be all of these aspects.

Willow: I'm very present to James Grotstein's book *Who Is The Dreamer Who Dreams The Dream?* (2000) in which he identified the *superordinate subject of being* and the *ineffable subject of the unconscious* or of the dream. He linked those two aspects of being, as *the dreamer who dreams the dream* (the superordinate subject of being) and the *dreamer who participates in the dream* or *the dreamer who experiences the dream*, or what he said was *the dreamer who understands the dream* (the ineffable subject of the unconscious), which he later amended as *participates in* with the nod to the fact that we never seal the dream (employing Freud's terms, there is always a *dream umbilicus*, even as there is also a *dream navel;* see Chapter 5).

The dream continues on in a sense that there's always a mystery to the dream, but that was the *ineffable subject of being of the unconscious* or of the dream. I loved how Grotstein, in that work, which has been so meaningful to me to learn and to study and be with, has been about ways of expanding the sense of Psyche. In reading Grotstein and in talking with him, I get the felt sense that Psyche is *everywhere* and *nowhere*—that she is *someone*, even as she is *anyone*. She is *everyone*. She is just *this one*. And, too, she is *no one*.

I think Psyche is all of those simultaneous presences and that's part of the grace of dreaming—that dreaming, as you say, dismantles our sense of self and other, our sense of subject-object, and in these really beautiful ways we are every aspect of the dream. At the same time, the dreamer who dreams the dream is mysterious and beyond self, beyond mind, beyond any graspability, any fixed identity.

Eva: There's something so haunting, almost that you were carried into this otherworldly, other historical experience, by participating and witnessing this ritual. There's something archetypal about it, and there is this incredible mystery. We don't necessarily know where or *why* Psyche took you there, *how* Psyche took you there. That always fills me with so much awe. What a gift that you just went to sleep and were given these, not just images, but also a real felt sense of participation.

Willow: Participation feels like the key dimension of the grace of dreaming, that dreaming is not just witnessing.

Eva: Right. It's not just watching a movie.

Willow: Yes. It's a felt sense that expands the felt sense of the one who experiences the dream, just as I feel it now sharing it with you. In this way, it is a conduit for experiential participation in emotional truth.

Eva: Again, I feel like, yes, your Psyche created the dream for you to enter, and now I'm getting to enter it with you. It touches me so much at this time of great divisiveness where people from two tribes are burying their dead. It reverberates in new ways. The dream is not, in other words, just for you, it's for everyone.

Willow: That feels like a meaningful part of the draw and inspiration and desire to write this book with you. Our dreams, even as they feel deeply personal, are, I believe, to be shared in sacred exchange in the manner in which we are invoking and participating in together.

Eva: I sense that is a lost art in our contemporary way of existing in the culture. This dream exchange could be happening in other cultures right now in ways I don't know about, which also has me thinking about, why turn our attention to the art of sharing dreams when there's so much upheaval and urgent political strife and violence and also an urgent Earth crisis?

Why should we invite our readers into this practice? Why is it important? You touched into that just now: We get to share in these experiences with each other and learn from them together and be in the dreamtime together. I don't necessarily have a clear answer to that question now, but it does feel one that's important to address: this practice isn't self-indulgence; it's not frivolous or naval gazing. There's something important to say about why dream sharing and dream practice is so relevant to today.

Willow: Perhaps more than "navel gazing" only—in other words, centered on more than the personal dimension of the dream—is also "umbilicus linking," which is tapped into the collective and, what's more, to cosmic consciousness. One of the things that comes to mind is that so much of the population is glued to the news cycle and how that is such a dominant narrative, globally, of our experience and meaning making. Psyche is the underground reporter, transmitting underground media about the ways in which we are deeply rooted together and the ways in which our fates are so inextricably bound and the ways in which our stories are so deeply rooted through matrices of interrelationship to one another, so beyond what we can grasp with our minds and with our current sense of separate identity.

That's one of the reasons that listening to, participating in, and sharing these sacred dreams feels vital at this time. It illustrates and demonstrates the ways in which we are bound to one another and expands our sense of identity to a more genuine understanding, a genuine recognition, where we are *someone* and *no one* and *anyone* and *everyone* and just *this one*.

Eva: That absolutely feels so true. It brings us into the realm of being participants in these living myths together. Dreaming is something that connects all humans. We all dream, no matter our ethnicity, our religion, all of these factors that can be so divisive. We are all dreaming creatures with hopes and longings and desires and fears and despairs.

As you're saying, there's something really essential now about touching into that shared humanity, that shared human experience, that we're all living through these mythic experiences. Your dream has a potent myth, as I hear it. Going into the dream feels like being taken into a myth or a … *folktale* is not quite the right word, but there's something timeless about the story that you shared and the experience of it.

Although I'm struggling to articulate my emotional truth, I hope you are following. We do need to get in touch with our emotional truth because, as you said, the news is so much about "us" versus "them" and "oppressed versus oppressor" and victimhood. It's taking us further away from the places that we share in our hopes and in our sorrows—we all bury our dead.

Willow: Relational psychoanalyst Jessica Benjamin's (2018) phrase of going beyond *doer and done to* captures the truth of Psyche because Psyche doesn't take sides. Psyche is all sides. Psyche invites us to participate in all dimensions and to move around our identification so it's not just with one tribe of self or experience. Psyche actually invites us to look at how, as you say, I'm both the one wrapping the corpses as well as the one who is the corpse.

Eva: The Great Spirit that is receiving corpses from both sides.

Willow: Yes. Indeed, from many sides.

Eva: In that sense, Psyche is really inviting us into a space where there's a shedding of certain skins that can keep us bounded into certain identities and certain stories of who we are. Often, people say, "I had this very strange dream," or "It was just so random," because that fluidity can feel hard for some people to explore or be open to.

A dream just ends up being labeled as sort of strange or fantastical. But if we can really allow ourselves to wonder about the dream and to wonder and freely associate with each of the elements that the dream is sharing and to invite others to do that as well, to me, that is when we enter sacred territory together. I do suspect some dreams are more conducive to or inviting of that wonderment than others.

This dream is about your ancestry, and there are particularities that I don't share in my own life, but the themes are universal. I wonder whether certain dreams are more sacred than other dreams—perhaps that's silly to even wonder—but I know in this project, we're being selective about the dreams that we're choosing to enter into …

Willow: There's something quite important about the dreams that call us. There are millions of dreams that I have. Last night, for instance, *I had a dream about a whole band of water skiers and my waterski went out, and I could only get half of it to work.* The dream felt vital and rich, and there was a lot there, but it's not a dream that I selected for our conversation or for the book because it didn't feel like a dream to draw back to the collective. It didn't feel like a dream with a call. (Yet, of course, at the same time and on another level, here I am invoking the dream, which seems to be about a whole that is reduced to half of itself, which is very on point with this dream of caesura's cry. And the water emanates as a metaphor for emotional life and access to it and so to emotional truth).

Eva: That makes sense. Is there anything else that lingers for you in the sharing of this particular dream that wants to come forth?

Willow: In looking up Île-à-la-Crosse, to learn more about its history as a geographic place, I also discovered that "The name Île-à-la-Crosse translated from French to English would be: Island of the Cross. The [European] name comes from the game La Crosse which was played by the [Indigenous] locals. When traders [of French Canadian and Scottish ancestry] arrived, they watched the [Indigenous people] play on Big Island and therefore named the place…Île-à-la-Crosse."[10] Further, the European naming of the region came from likening the shape of the area lake to a Bishop's stick or crosse.[11]

Eva: Yeah, I was definitely taken by the name of the place. Obviously in English, we know *cross*, and also symbolically we have the sense of *coming to a crossroads* (Eva holds up her wrists to the video camera and interlocks them, for me to see her dynamic gesture) or the two different directions and the two different ancestral lineages coming to this place and linking the two different tribes. That felt important, that the dream situated you in this particular geography.

Willow: I mean, just to close at this moment, when you make that gesture with your interlocking wrists, it portends for me a symbol of the crossing of heaven and earth.

Eva: Between the material and the spirit realms.

Willow: Yes. Thank you for receiving and engaging this stream with me today.

Eva: Thank you. It feels like a particular balm that is needed, a salve that is needed for me right now. Even as I'm sitting in front of bright blue skies and these beautiful oak trees, there is this heaviness that I spoke to in the beginning of our conversation of just knowing there's so much suffering happening on the planet at this time of war and your sharing this dream with me. It is the balm. It is a medicine that provides some important solace for me at this time.

Willow: Thank you, Eva.

Apprenticing Grace in the Afterward: Dream Blessing

As I write now, on September 13, 2024, I am struck by how this dream teaches me to apprentice Grace, in apprenticing a given dream. In particular, I am struck by the unfolding of blessing. I only now realize, a year after receiving this nighttime dream, that I received a wedding gift from my dear friend Nina Farana that carried her blessing and the blessing of the Zuni people of New Mexico.

Nina, a dear friend who I met at Stanford University when I was an undergraduate, is a devout Catholic who creates incredibly beautiful hand-crafted collages of sacred iconography. She has many artworks devoted to Mary and to Christ. I treasure and so deeply value her art that my family collectively purchased one of her pieces, a work of Mary, to gift my mother-in-law for Christmas, 2023. Nina is also a poet (hear "Roar," a song from my first album, *Burning*, 2002; the lyrics of Roar are of two poems authored by Nina).

Nina was unable to attend our wedding, in 2022, in person. In her stead, she sent us a most treasured card and gift. I quote from the card, with Nina's permission:

> July 2022
>
> Willow and Daniel:
>
> I pray you had a beautiful day on the 18th and that whatever depth of love you had experienced together before that date grows deeper still now that it has been annunciated as a sacred bond. I apologize for the lateness of this note. I have been wondering what to send you both to mark the day. It finally came to me to send you two little guardians for your journey. There is a lovely tradition among the Zuni people here of carving animal fetishes. Each has its own meaning and magic. I chose an otter for you—the bearer of laughter, curiosity, grace and empathy—and also a songbird. The symbolism of the latter, I think, will be obvious. In any event, a messenger of heaven and a creature that rolls with the waves seemed to me good reminders of how to respond to the ups and downs of any relationship. The dust on both of these is from cornmeal which has been sprinkled on each as a blessing. They come to you bearing my very best wishes to you. It is good to be together. Cherish each other. Love. Laugh. Pray.
>
> Nina

So, a year after receiving the dream, I realize that Nina's blessing, containing the Zuni blessings, taught me something about the Indigenous soul that appeared in my dream, wrapping the bodies of the dead in deerskin blankets (the Zuni animal fetishes arrived wrapped in deerskin pouches—one was pale green, wrapping the otter, and the other one was a warm tan color, for the songbird) and sprinkling them with cornmeal. And in apprenticing the dream, I am apprenticing Grace, here in the nested forms of a dream blessing, born of Catholic and Indigenous (Metís-Cree and Zuni) lineages.

Eva and I had our dream dialogue in late October, 2023. We could barely speak about and name the atrocities endured by Israel and Gaza, tearing at our souls and the souls of so many, even as that war's emergence was omnipresent in the dream field between us and is raging still, claiming the lives of an untold number of souls.[12]

In these ways, the dream medicine was ministered equally to the past, the present, and the future, on personal and collective levels at once. That recognition itself is a dream blessing born of apprenticing Grace, offered here to you, the reader. May the dream medicine be yours too, and may it travel further still, as a giveaway.

Notes

1 For context on Charlotte Small Thompson, a Metís-Cree woman, and her marriage to David Thompson, an Englishman who immigrated to Canada, see Pearson Trimbach (2022).
2 See "Île-à-la-Crosse," Wikipedia, https://en.wikipedia.org/wiki/%C3%8Ele-%C3%A0-la-Crosse
3 See Eshel (2022) for an invocation of "Perhaps a Cry for a Caesura?" where I first heard/read/considered this poignant expression of "caesura's cry." See also Pearson Trimbach (2025)—an album of original songs entitled *Caesura's Cry*.
4 See "Meet Île-à-la-Crosse," *Sakitawak Conservation*, https://sakitawakconservation.wordpress.com/meet-ile-a-la-crosse/
5 See also Île-à-la-Crosse, Wikipedia, https://en.wikipedia.org/wiki/%C3%8Ele-%C3%A0-la-Crosse
6 See "Meet Île-à-la-Crosse."
7 See Michael Eigen's work on distinction-union, which I am centering here as an expression of the caesura. See Grotstein and Pearson (2016) and Pearson (2021) for a discussion of the psychoanalytic term *caesura*. See Pearson (2021) for reflections on caesuras of dreaming and Trimbach (2022) for a practice of dreaming the caesura.
8 For an overview of Metis-Cree death ceremonies and rituals, including wrapping the coffins of the deceased with material, see Barkwell (n.d.). For a discussion of the historical mourning practices of the Cree and Ojibway, including "providing the corpse with necessary items for the spirit's journey to the afterlife," see Hackett (2005).
9 Robin Bagai, Toxic Nourishment Seminar, February 4, 2024. Used with permission from *RobinBagai.com*
10 See "Meet Île-à-la-Crosse."
11 See D. McLennan, "Île-à-la-Crosse," https://www.esask.uregina.ca/tmc_cms/modules/customcode/includes/print_entry.cfm-entryid=734B4EEA-1560-95DA-433708767408FBB0.html
12 Transgenerational trauma (Salberg & Grand, 2024, 2017a, 2017b) centers the conversation. Listening for caesura's cry (Eshel, 2022) serves as catalyst for, container for, and commentary on dreaming a "new Île-à-la-Crosse." "War as a means of cross-fertilization" is invoked (personal communication, Michael Eigen online seminar, April 30, 2024).

References

Barkwell, L. (n.d.). *Metis culture: Metis death rituals and ceremonies*. Gabriel Dumont Institute, Virtual Museum of Metis History and Culture. https://www.metismuseum.ca/media/document.php/11728.Metis%20Death%20Ceremonies.pdf

Benjamin, J. (2018). *Beyond doer and done to: Recognition theory, intersubjectivity and the third*. Routledge.

Eshel, O. (2022). Bion's long road toward intuiting the patient's suffering: "Theoretical" vs. "clinical" Bion. *Contemporary Psychoanalysis*, *58*(1), 46–76. https://doi.org/10.1080/00107530.2022.2083424

Grotstein, J. (2000). *Who is the dreamer, who dreams the dream?* The Analytic Press.

Grotstein, J., & Pearson, W. (2016). In conversation on caesura and reversible perspective. *Fort Da: The Journal of the Northern California Society for Psychoanalytic Psychology*, *22*(1), 51–60.

Hackett, P. (2005). Historical mourning practices observed among the Cree and Ojibway Indians of the Central Subarctic. *Ethnohistory*, *52*, 503–532. https://doi.org/10.1215/00141801-52-3-503

Macdougall, B. (2010). *One of the family: Metis culture in nineteenth-century northwestern Saskatchewan*. University of British Columbia Press.

Pearson, W. (2021). Caesuras of dreaming: Being and becoming, thinking and imagining. In W. Pearson & H. Marlo (Eds.), *The spiritual psyche: Mysticism, intersubjectivity, and psychoanalysis* (pp. 180–201). Routledge.

Pearson Trimbach, W. (2025). Caesura's cry [Audio recording]. Retrieved from https://www.lionessroars.org/music/caesuras-cry

Pearson Trimbach, W. (2022). Integral relational practice of dreaming the caesura. Part 1: Opening further through the spiritual psyche. Part 2: Dreaming Charlotte Small Thompson. *Jung Journal: Culture & Psyche*, *16*(4), 115–123.

Salberg, J., & Grand, S. (Eds.). (2017a). *Trans-generational trauma and the Other: Dialogues across history and difference*. Routledge.

Salberg, J., & Grand, S. (Eds.). (2017b). *Wounds of history: Repair and resilience in the trans-generational transmission of trauma*. Routledge.

Salberg, J., & Grand, S. (2024). *Transgenerational trauma: A contemporary introduction*. Routledge.

12
ASCENSION
Learning from Divinity

Memoir of the Future[1]

I wrote the following prequel in 2020 at the time of sharing the nighttime dream presented here. I did not yet imagine asking Eva to coauthor this book with me. Yet, clearly, the inspiration to cowrite the book was seeded on this very occasion of giving voice to this "Ascension: Learning from Divinity" dream. In 2023, the idea of co-writing this book with Eva was given to me in a dream. Yet, I can see now, apparently, that 2023 dream of co-authorship was nested in the 2020 dream that follows.

Prequel: 2020 Chuppah Dreams in a Garden of Eden

The night of April 25, 2020, I had a most beautiful, compelling, and vivid dream. As I sit to write about the dream, I realize this dream appeared exactly three months to the day following my only brother's death on January 25, 2020, at just fifty years old. The dream appeared the night before I was to "gather (virtually) in the Garden of Eden" with dear friends Adam and Eva, as their kind invitation was named—an invitation to meet on Zoom with other dear friends of theirs, just one month into COVID lockdown. I first spoke about the following dream in that Garden of friendship, on April 26, 2020. At the time, I did not realize the waking dream of the chuppah through which I met two friends of Adam and Eva, another couple, via Zoom. Yet the chuppah of Eva and Adam's love held me. Adam and Eva had invited the five of us each to speak about the topic of perspective at this moment of lockdown, and I chose to share about how dreaming, and the myriad perspectives it can engender, is a constant companion and contemplation for me. I did not fully intend to share the following dream that I had the night before. But as I began speaking, it seemed that the container of the virtual Garden of Eden, that chuppah,

DOI: 10.4324/9781003591863-13

allowed my previous night's dream to emerge and begin to show its face, or at least its outline.

At the time, I did not share the initial working title for my book in progress, *The Grace of Dreaming* (later to become *The Emotional Truth of Dreams*). So it was a sweet synchronicity, indeed, when this couple announced the name of their unborn daughter, Grace. I realized in that moment that the three of us would all be on a dedicated path of learning about Grace, from the ground of creative inception and devotion—they about their daughter as she came into being and I about this book, a different kind of creative emergence, requiring a kindred spirit, tending, opening into mystery, and daily learning for years to come.

Certainly, receiving this dream was a grace. The dream is about Christ's ascension. Given the fact that I was not raised in a religious faith, the dream is all the more compelling to me. (Ours was a seemingly secular home—my father was a molecular geneticist and my mother was a social worker, yet theirs was a devotion to science and a devotion to social services born of great compassion.) Although at the time of this writing, I have been teaching at a Catholic University for the past three years and I am now in partnership with a devoted Catholic man (for more than a year now), and although I attended a Friends (Quaker) school from the eighth grade to my senior year of high school and practiced Meeting for Worship in the Quaker tradition, I have never formally studied the Christian tradition. My spiritual and religious study has centered on Tibetan Buddhism for most of my adult life. Rather, I have considered myself a kindred mystic with curiosity about how my own experience of faith and spirit also draws from many different traditions, including the Christian and Jewish traditions that I have not formally studied or religiously practiced. Growing up, I have celebrated a mostly secular version of Christmas and Easter centered, not on the church, but on family bonds. In recent years, I have wanted to learn more about mystical and progressive Christianity, so I ordered two books that now live on my shelf: *Resurrecting Jesus* by Adyashanti (2016) and *Finding Jesus at the Border* by high-school friend and California Lutheran Associate Professor Julia Lambert Fogg (2020).

Finding Jesus at the Border literally arrived on April 25, the day of the Zoom gathering. Both books have yet to be opened and read.

In the Dream....

In the dream, Jesus has risen, ascended to the beyond that has no beginning and no end, no destination and no absence of place. He has ascended to a place of everywhere and nowhere that is somewhere just beyond here and yet dwells too in this very place. He just departed. But so many were present for, yet did not behold, his passage to the "upper room." Instead, they ended their observance with his crucifixion. But that was a path of human sorrow that did not end there.

In an attempt to convey something of the majesty of Christ's ascension, people were building a living sculpture across several interconnected art installations that depicted multiple aspects of Christ's life, messages, and teachings. The project would take years to complete and was already underway.

I was responsible for a secular fresco. It was a tribute to Jane. In the dream, Jane was a feminist of renown who was to be remembered and so memorialized in the context of Christ's field. The location of this fresco was toward the middle of the living sculpture. Even so, people could easily miss it. In the dream, my first-grade teacher was kind enough to meet with me to help me get the details of Jane's life correct for the art installation. In the dream, the entire installation was at the front of my former high school, Wilmington Friends School, such that the entrance was transformed into this living story of Christ's ascension. There was a question as to whether the installation would be white marble or sandstone, painted in gold leaf and color. I hoped it would be painted sandstone, in living color.

There was another installation just to the right of Jane's and up the hill. It was Hercules's installation. And so many were drawn there who did not understand the relationships among Christ, Hercules, and Jane and so could not behold them as part of an interwoven storyboard, thinking of them instead as entirely separate art pieces divorced from one another. I looked forward to the day that the art installations would be complete and art-goers would be able to take in the stories and their links to one another.

There were tourists milling though the frescos and the art installations, even as they were under construction. I was very proud of etching the first drawing of Jane's feminist memorial on the sandstone. (As I write this now, I think of Jane Leland Stanford and her creation of the Stanford Memorial Church, in sandstone and gold leaf and color, which I so admired and sought refuge in as an undergraduate.) *The etching was barely discernible to the passersby. But I could make it out. The work had begun to take shape. The first marks had been made.*

As I write this now, I think of this dream as the beginning of the book, with its working title of *The Grace of Dreaming*, the first marks on the page, the beginning outline of a barely perceptible shape. What stands out is the vast majesty of Christ's ascension, which animates the whole field and yet which, paradoxically, so few people are conscious of. *In the dream, I am able to take both perspectives—the perspective of one who beholds Christ's ascension and the perspective of one who does not have access to that part of Christ's story.*

Postscript: 2020 Pointing Out Grace

I am beginning, in writing this book, an apprenticeship to Grace. She has, I now imagine, always been with me but I have not known her well by her name.

I am reminded of a Freudian slip that I made just the other day when talking with my colleague, Helen Marlo. She was asking about my Zoom subscription. And mishearing her, I repeated back a shocking question, "I am going to be exhumed?!" This was the day after Easter and a client had talked to me that very afternoon about his sorrow that so many people were dying alone in this COVID-19 crisis. I was trying to put together who or what accompanies us when we die. I was thinking about Christ's resurrection. And I was wondering if Christ is there to accompany people when they die. Or who or what might be. I suppose a part of me was identifying with my brother, being exhumed from the earth and from the body and feeling the bewilderment of "What now?" I would like to think that Grace accompanies him, then and now.

Perhaps, the fresco memorializing Jane is a tribute to Grace in secular form? Perhaps this is my piece of the story to write and to live out.

I remember performing U2's song "Grace" with my band in Boulder, Colorado, in the early 2000s. I will have to give the song another listen. Beginning my conscious apprenticeship as I write my first pages of this book on *The Grace of Dreaming*, I wish to tune my ears and, indeed, my psyche to Grace.

In the Afterward of Ascension: 2024

Willow: I welcome any reveries, associations, wonderments, links that come into your heart and mind in hearing this expression of the prequel, the dream, and the postscript.

Eva: There are so many different places to approach the dream. I want to enter into the triangle though—between Hercules, Christ, and Jane. These archetypes feel so powerful, especially because you don't have, as you revealed, a specific relationship to Christ, as I don't either, I should disclose. I believe that allows our imaginations to expand around the figure of Christ precisely because we don't have one particular meaning associated with Christ and his ascension. And I'm, of course, most drawn to Jane, the feminist secular artist—perhaps because that archetype feels closest to home …

Willow: Yes, Jane, the secular artist, is the archetype in the dream that feels closest to home for both of us. And yet, the trio, the triangle they compose, is the central archetype of the dream …

Eva: That line where you said Jane's part of the fresco was in the center of this larger installation, but "it would be easy to miss" or "people could easily miss it," really hit me in a particular way. Throughout so much of history women have been creating—whether through their minds or through their spirits or through their hands or all of those channels—yet how easy it has been for history to miss those creations, perhaps in juxtaposition to Herculean efforts, which are characteristically bold, forceful, and masculine. I'm curious how you're relating to this triangle, how these three dream energies coalesce for you?

Willow: What's interesting is the dream gave me the vivid sense of their union, the union of the triangle, within me. The dream was like a living, felt understanding of my deep connection to Hercules, the strong man, and of Christ and his story not ending with his death, and the interdependence of the three of us.

And also the yearning for the art-goers, the tourists, to make the connections between these storyboards of the art installation—the fresco and the other pieces—in the way that these three beings, these archetypes—artists of spirit, artists of materiality, and artists of creation—are inextricably linked.

Eva: Yes. I think we could say that Christ is the spirit that transcends and Hercules is of the body.

Willow: Yes, Hercules is of the earth.

Eva: And then Jane perhaps is the union between the two, where the heart resides.

Willow: She's very much the medium between the two…

And that Jane the dream figure, in the form of Jane Leland Stanford, literally created the temple of the Stanford Memorial Church, the place on the Stanford campus that I sought refuge in as an undergraduate. It was actually the first physical place that I connected to on campus, and it was my presence there in the church that made me know that I wanted to attend Stanford. I had made a journey from Delaware on the East Coast, where I was living at age eighteen, to a presentation by Yolanda King, Dr. Martin Luther King's daughter. Her presentation was delivered on Martin Luther King Day in Memorial Church. And so I flew there to hear her speak, and Memorial Church was the very first building that I entered on the Stanford campus. Her speaking there had a huge impact on me, as did the quotes that select church sandstones are painted with.

I remember my visit there on that threshold occasion bringing me a sense of connection. It showed up in my dream as the union of the creativity of these quotes and the artistry of the church itself and the beauty of the architecture, together with it being a house of spirit, which again is striking for me as someone who grew up in a secular household. And it was not in any way incidental that a dream of Christ entered my psyche through union with Daniel, my husband, and union with Notre Dame de Namur University (NDNU), where I was teaching at the time, and literally visited me in a way that I could feel and know on the interior where I had not had, as we said, any particular conscious previous personal relationship to Christ. And that dream gave me a point of felt access, of personal access, a direct link to Christ. And in many ways, it came through my being at NDNU and my relationship with Daniel, both of which obviously have a very, very strong connection in their Catholic tradition to Christ.

Eva: It's so beautiful that the dream could be a portal for you to have a felt sense of intimacy with this historical figure, but also this archetypal energy, and that it's not something that you could just read about in a book and have an intellectual sense of Christ as being and as archetype. When we talk about the emotional truth of dreams, this was an emotional truth of relatedness to the spirit, the being, the archetype of Christ, that you could only immediately experience through the dream.

Willow: I'm touched by both of those books on Jesus by Adyashanti and Julia Lambert Fogg, the ones that I have on my bookshelf, but the only reading I've done is of this dream. This dream is what brings me a sense of felt and direct connection, and I want to say it is trustable in that sense, faithful in that sense to emotional truth. I wasn't instructed to do something. The dream came unbidden.

Eva: For me, that is also where the feminine, Jane and the creative artist, comes in because it's trusting the feminine path of knowing, of creativity. It's not something that has just been externally given to you or taught to you, and then you're supposed to take in that knowledge as truth with a capital *T,* right? The dream itself is this very artistic experience. You are wandering this installation and feeling this sense of wonder. Psyche created this very beautiful artistic landscape for you to have, as you said, a direct experience of this spiritual energy.

Willow: As you say that, what comes through even more strongly by sharing the dream is the other emotional truth of the dream—when we die, we ascend. I understand that's a religious teaching, but it's not a religious teaching that I grew up with. It's not an understanding that I've studied or followed, you could say, from a Christian reference point. And again, from the perspective of the dream, which I can touch in this moment, the perspective of the dream was utter clarity that yes, Christ died, but also he ascended. And there was a clarity, by extension, that is the truth of spirit, that we leave the body and we continue. And I know that there are many faiths and many orientations about what that might mean or look like or be like or how it might be held—all of that is beyond the scope of the dream. But that very simple direct feeling, the emotional truth of the dream was very clear—that when Christ died, his life wasn't over. And the sharing of this dream revelation was opened into through the chuppah of love between you and Adam, at a time of social isolation for all of us. In a parallel of being, the arc of your love and union with Adam created a bridge between transcendence and immanence, to celestial presence through the terrestrial presence, indivisible, as welcoming and as guide.

Eva: I'm appreciative, if I have the timeline correct in my mind, that we could also see this as a grief dream. This dream arose in the wake of mourning your brother' disappearance, which was also in the wake of entering into COVID lockdown. I don't think I put that together, that he had passed just three months prior to the dream, in January, 2020. And so to be in that place of private grief, but then to have the world open up into this place of more collective fragility and vulnerability … I wonder if you can speak to the dream as an expression of grieving on this journey.

Willow: Absolutely. As I wrote in the postscript, I was really reflecting on my brother Scott's death. At that time, in a way that was prescient and in a way that is present for mourners after the loss of a loved one in a more acute way than usual (as I'm sure you must feel, too, with the loss of your mentor/teacher recently), was this living sense of "Where did he go? How was he accompanied?" It wasn't a formulated question so much as a felt wonder.

I think those two questions are what it comes down to for me. Where did he go? How was he accompanied? And in a way in this moment, I can say, "Well, it's very clear where he lives is in my heart and the heart of all the friends and family members who cherish him." That could be one place. And he's also accompanied by all of us who cherish him in our expressions of loss and reverie. Those expressions accompany him in some way. And there may be other answers to those questions as well that are beyond me, but those are the ones that the dream presences in the telling of it now. Those are the emotional truths of telling you the dream and relating it now.

Eva: Thank you. That really resonates. Are there other places that you want to explore within the dreamscape?

Willow: Just appreciating these multiple covalent, mutually arising themes of the dream of my brother's death; of the mediumship of feminist creative midwifery; of Christ's life, death, and ascension; and the triangle of archetypes. And the last one I'll add is the reading of this dream through the chuppah of union between you and Adam that then held and that also now continues to hold space for the furthering of our dream incubations. As the opening into our book and the first marks on the page, it feels so clear how your invitation to that Zoom gathering during COVID lockdown allowed me to speak the dream and share it with you in a way that brought it into relationship with you and into the world. I don't know if or when it may have come into expression otherwise, if not for your and Adam's invitation to "gather in the Garden of Eden."

Eva: I am so grateful that we created that container so that this dream could have a place of holding and witnessing. And I do think it feels right, this triangle of spirit, body, and heart—transcendence, immanence, and the dance between the two, which is Jane's work as the creative artist. What a strong triangle that psyche brought forth. It opens us into so much of what this book is about.

Willow: What's striking to me also about the dream, just to repeat what I've already said, is that in the dream, the embrace and living understanding of that triangle, that trinity, was already present as opposed to being a dream that was about trying to weave that together or trying to bring that to life. There was a desire to share that and transmit that through the completion of the art installation and the invitation of the art-goers. In that sense, we could regard the dream art installation itself as a kind of collective chuppah—a kind of spiritual canopy—uniting Jane, Hercules, Christ, and the art-goers. The dream itself was a vision, a living truth that I don't always feel the integration of in my daily life, not in the way that I felt in the dream. In the dream, there was utter confluence. There was no obstacle, no barrier to the link of that triad, of that trinity of Jane the creative artist, Hercules the strong man, and Christ the ascendent spirit. And a further opening to the convergent quartet of Jane, Hercules, Christ, and the art-goers, through the sheltering ephemeral-yet-palpable chuppah.

Note

1 Here I invoke the title of Bion's (1991) book. A beautiful example of *A Memoir of the Future* is Eva's (2024) luminous book, *Bodywork*, which includes images from a forgotten archive of her artwork, created a decade prior to the onset of a debilitating illness uncannily forecast in these images. For a stunning review of Eva's book, see https://www.birchbarkediting.com/microlit-almanac-reviews/bodywqork-eva-tuschman-leonard-marsha-recknagel

References

Adyashanti. (2016). *Resurrecting Jesus*. Sounds True.
Bion, W. R. (1991). *A memoir of the future*. Karnac.
Lambert Fogg, J. (2020). *Finding Jesus at the border*. Brazos Press.
Tuschman Leonard, E. T. (2024). *Bodywork*. Bored Wolves.

13

GRACE

Learning from Living—Tara's Promise

Presencing music as dreaming,[1] this chapter demonstrates dreaming as original artistry through the soul's emergence as song (Pearson, 2021). Music as an actualization of and metaphor for dreaming life is expressed through contemplation of the verses of "Tara's Promise," a song from Willow's original music catalogue, as the Watermoons, dedicated to the Noble Lady Tara. We explore the relationship between the Buddhist deity Tara and the universal revelations of grace as moments of opening to the soul and as paths of liberation, supported by Jung's synchronicity (Marlo, 2022). Willow's nighttime dream of Eva, an expression of the spiritual psyche (Pearson & Marlo, 2021), figures *dreaming soul* and *touching grace.* Dreaming this demonstrates and transmits Tara's "appearance–emptiness–appearance," "sound–emptiness–sound," and the "clarity–emptiness–thought" of co-dreaming (Haq & Masih, 2018), through nested dreams, dreaming's reach, and the simulcast of dreams. In this way, honoring the mystery of the soul, the grace of dreaming, in learning from living, is realized as none other than the dreaming of Grace as Tara.

~~~

Upon waking, I once again reflect on the sense that "Our dreams are closer than our eyes. They are sustained and revealed in love. This is why sometimes we cannot see them."

Here is the dream from which that reflection arose …

Dreaming's Reach

5/14/24

I dream that at 6 o'clock Eva will take leave and at 7 o'clock people will not be able to study their dreams with her.

DOI: 10.4324/9781003591863-14
~~~

I awaken and speak this out loud, mostly still asleep, in distress to my husband. What can I do to make it possible for Eva to teach on dreams with the 7 o'clock group?

I go back to sleep and have the same dream again.

I awaken thinking that this is a dream that looks backward and forward at once, from the present, and is a source of possible birth of Eva's dream communication.

In a sense, the dream asks, how can this teaching on dreaming live on, beyond our presence on Earth? In response, this dream called forth a song entitled "Tara's Promise," which I wrote with my music partner Eric Ramstad, as The Watermoons, in 2012.

Tara is a central Buddhist deity of enlightenment and compassion. Her promise is to be ever-present, to always be reachable, and, equally, to return to Earth again and again to help human beings. Eva calls Tara to mind, and in that spirit, here are my interpretations of the song "Tara's Promise"[2] in the light of *dreaming's reach.* As I have written elsewhere, dreaming is a form of original artistry (Pearson, 2021; Polit Dillon, 2024). Here I am holding this song, "Tara's Promise," itself as a dream. And so this very writing, inspired by dreaming Eva, which in turn inspired "Tara's Promise," is an experience of a nested dream within a dream within a dream. … As I will uncover, the relationship between the Buddhist deity Tara and the universal revelations of grace as moments of opening to the soul and as paths of liberation, are presenced by my dream of Eva, which is supported by Jung's synchronicity (Marlo, 2022).

Tara's Promise[3]

Music by The Watermoons, lyrics by Willow Pearson
Recorded on The Watermoons' first album, *Red Boat*

Om tare tutare ture soha[4]
Om tare tu tare ture soha
Om tare tu tare ture soha
Om tare tu tare ture soha

I will travel with you
until you get by
Prajnaparamita
into the night

rest in the openness
and lend your sight
to every being
in this delight

steady your gaze
kiss the sky
unfurl the waves

and ride…
and ride…

Om tare tutare ture soha
Om tare tutare ture soha

look into the mirror
nothing shall arise
pray beyond hope and fear
this is how to fly

give your love
give your love away
and so discover
that it wears another face

steady your gaze
kiss the sky
unfurl the waves
and ride…
and ride…

Om tare tutare ture soha
Om tare tutare ture soha

in your emerald sky palace
light streams in
from all sides
and in the openness
the searching heart will oblige

the three jewels
adorn your heart
as peace beyond suffering
you make your mark
with your eyes of moon and sun
in your celestial home
there's room for everyone

steady your gaze
kiss the sky
unfurl the waves
and ride…
and ride…

Om tare tutare ture soha
Om tare tutare ture soha
Om tare tutare ture soha
Om tare tutare ture soha
Om tare tutare ture soha

The song begins with a fourfold prayer to Lady Tara, the deity of great compassion, the mother of all Buddhas, the feminine divine in her immanent and transcendent myriad forms. In this way, the traditional homage, supplication, aspiration, and request that open all Buddhist teachings are contained within and invoked by Tara's mantra: *Om tare tutare ture soha.* Tara, we pay homage to you, our Liberator, our savioress. *Om tare tutare ture soha.* Tara, we supplicate you, to bless us with your presence at this very moment and to be with us always. *Om tare tutare ture soha.* Tara, we aspire to follow your example and to realize your teachings of great compassion. *Om tare tutare ture soha.* Tara, we request you turn the wheel of dharma and teach us in this very moment, right here, on the spot.

I will travel with you
until you get by
Prajnaparamita
into the night

Tara is saying, "I will never leave you. I will always be here for you." And "Prajnaparamita / into the night" is perhaps the most potent, pith phrase in the entire *Red Boat* song cycle (Watermoons, 2012). *Prajnaparamita* is the great *Yum Chenmo*, the origin point of no origin, the void that is always pregnant, the original face of emergence that is paradoxically "before" and yet also contiguous with any appearance. She may be designated as "O" in psychoanalytic streams—Bion's symbol for the unknown, unknowable emotional truth of a therapeutic session—or a twin sister perhaps. Prajnaparamita is that essential drop from which all forms, all appearances in their sacred and profane guises—within, between, and among us—take shape. So, Prajnaparamita as Tara manifests as the birthplace of the movement of consciousness in gross, subtle, causal, and nondual ways, as we might say in integral terms. Or Prajnaparamita as Tara manifests in *nirmanakaya* (gross body), *sambogakaya* (subtle body), dharmakaya (*transcendent body*), and *svavaikakaya* (integral body) embodiments, as we might say in the Buddhist lineage. She wears all of these appearances.

"Prajnaparamita / into the night": In the darkest place of the unknown and the unknowable, Tara *is* with us. She is that benevolent force. Tara demonstrates that the Good is never not present.

rest in the openness
and lend your sight

through every being
in this delight

Rest in the openness. "Rest" is the pith instruction. Rest in the openness. Rest in the awareness. Relax and let go. And lend your sight. What does that mean? It is a supplication to Tara, a request for Tara to lend her guidance to this wandering being, this listener, this supplicator. It is also a request *from* Tara. "You, my student, my devotee, that one whom I protect, lend your sight. Open your eyes. Bring your unique self, your unique perspective, to this occasion. Summon your clarity and bring it forth." Furthermore, this line carries these twin injunctions to underscore, "in this delight": "Rest in the openness / and lend your sight / through every being / in this delight." Lend your sight to every being. Involve as many perspectives as you possibly can in the expanse of your heart and mind. And do come through with your unique perspective, right within that expanse. Don't fail to come through with your voice. At the right moment. At the right time. With your right speech. In this delight. This is the way in which you are both a participant in the whole, a manifestation of the whole, and a vessel for the whole. You are receiver; you are conduit; you are witness. And you are *that*. All of it. Nothing at all is quite something.

steady your gaze
kiss the sky
unfurl the waves
and ride…
and ride…

"Steady your gaze" the song exhorts in the chorus. "Kiss the sky." So in the yogic traditions, *Drishti*, or the gaze, is extremely important. On the level of physical practice, of life's asana practice, the continual threading of yogic poses, Drishti is how we steady our self-understanding of what we are doing, of why we are here, how we give our attention to what is of importance. This line underscores the need for concentration, the need for focus. And in that steadying of the gaze, the simultaneous instruction contained in the song is "kiss the sky." So right within that focus of selected attention is the yogic exhortation of awareness to be available for the expanse, to be aware of both figure and ground, however we continue to practice that in our endeavors. "Unfurl the wave. In this delight …" There is instruction here on navigating the karmic knot, the endless knot, whatever the difficulty is that we are facing in the moment, whatever ripple we are riding that can take us off balance if we fight against it trying to stay still. How do we move with that wave? "Unfurl the wave … in this delight." This karmic activity is ceaseless, is without end. And so, if you are not delighting now, when? Enjoy as you go!

look into the mirror
nothing shall arise

pray beyond hope and fear
this is how to fly

"Look into the mirror / nothing shall arise." These lines are embracing that paradox, the simplicity on the other side of complexity. "Look into the mirror." See everything as a sacred mirror. Behold everything as self / no-self: the within, the between, and the among—first, second, and third person. The *within* is the *I*. The *between, I-thou*. And *among*, the *third person*. And *around*, the *third person*. See everything as a reflection of the mirror mind, the mind that contains body, mind, and spirit. *Dharmakaya*—that which contains everything. "Look into the mirror / nothing shall arise." There is a uniformity, a union, a sameness, an every-ness, an all-ness. In a sense, nothing shall arise. There is nothing to arise. There is no other. And nothing *shall* arise. That emptiness shall appear. That emptiness is not merely empty. That appearance–emptiness–appearance will shine as luminosity.

In the second half of the stanza, "Pray beyond hope and fear / this is how to fly." Here the traditional instruction, teaching, and wisdom that is impossible to miss in the Buddhist lineage is invoked: be available for that which is beyond hope and fear. The song points us toward the great middle way. The mind is habitually caught in thoughts and wishes, fantasies and projections of hope and fear, of attraction and aversion. Still, what else is available to awareness when we pull back from, or just look straight into, those facets of mind?

This is how to fly.

The other traditional teaching that is hard to miss is invoked through the song by flight. The song here points to the *dakas* and *dakinis*—angels in Western cosmology—the spiritual beings we can hold in awareness as self and other, and also as the transcendent, ethereal communications from the sky beings that visit us on the top of our head, that visit us straight like an arrow into the heart, that visit us in every bodily center and energy channel that runs through us. Every *nadi*, every movement of mind, every delusion. Everything. The song entreats us to pray beyond hope and fear. Pray, the song pleads, that you will touch awareness that is beyond hope and fear. Mind you that awareness doesn't have to exclude hope and fear, but it also contacts that dimension of mind that is beyond hope and fear and not trapped by them, not reduced to them. This is how to fly. This is how Tara flies. This is how she moves through the three times. This is how she moves through the inseparability of past, present, and future. This is how the dakas and dakinis move. This is how the deities move. This is how they move. Adyashanti (2025) always asks, "How does It move?" I might elaborate on this query by adding, "How does spirit move in you, as you, through you? How does spirit move?" The song is teaching us if we are paying attention: *this* is how it moves. *This* is how Tara flies.

give your love
give your love away

and so discover
that it wears another face

There is a wonderful line in a book by David Whyte called *Pilgrim* (Whyte, 2012), that says "the ultimate purification is to love and to let go." And these song lines are, to my heart, another way of saying just that. "Give your love / give your love away / and so discover / that it wears another face." By loving and letting go, we discover the essence of love. We learn something about the nature of love. We learn that in the act of loving we are expanded (in spite of and in response to our contractions). These lines are an expression of the core Buddhist teaching on nonattachment. They cut through the confusion about that teaching … hopefully, by clarifying that nonattachment is not about isolation, it's not about withholding, it's not about defending—although we certainly do all of those things and we need not castigate ourselves for that. Yet, love is something that we give away because we cannot ever know its effect really. Even on ourselves, we scarcely know love's effect, really, as the bounds of love are always greater than what we can apprehend in conscious awareness.

So, give your love. Give it away. Don't be attached to the outcome. And so discover that it wears another face. And what face is that? We discover that we are Tara, that we wear her face, in the act of loving and letting go. That she is truly, as we suspected, inseparable from us, when we catch a glimpse of her in action through us. We discover firsthand that we do love bigger than ourselves. That is actually the nature of love. What other face do we discover that love wears? We discover, of course, that it is the beloved; it is the one whom we give our love to. Tara is that one as well, that beloved.

This song was conceived at the onset of a beautiful and challenging relationship between me and co-songwriter Eric Ramstad—a gifted guitar player, producer, and arranger. The creation of this song and its production also marks the beginning, middle, and indeed the end, the after-end, and the continuation of our friendship. Through this song, both of us were called to the mat again and again, called to our seat again and again, to give our love away and discover that it wears another face. That love, that Tara, wears the face of ourselves, surprisingly, at moments. We discovered, in glances and glimpses, how love, how Tara, wears the face of the other, quite beautifully. Ultimately, we discovered how love, how Tara, appears in the music itself. We learned that the music itself is a *sambogakaya* (subtle body) appearance of Tara, distinct from and yet no other than who we actually are.

steady your gaze
kiss the sky
unfurl the waves
and ride…
and ride…

Here again, the chorus is teaching us how to do that, how to pray beyond hope and fear. How to fly? Steady your gaze. On the mat. On the yoga mat. In asana practice. Literally on the cushion in meditation. Formally. Literally in post-meditation, in daily life. In the dreamtime. Steady your gaze, kiss the sky. Focus and release. Discipline and freedom. Engage expansively. Look at what's right here and now and the context in which that is happening. Center and edge.

Unfurl the waves in this delight. When you're bunched up, smooth it out as best you can. Know that the wave is the water, inseparable, as best you can. And touch bliss in this. Realize that the delight is not tomorrow. Or yesterday. Don't wait for the delight. Let it be right here, right now. In *this* delight.

in your emerald sky palace
light streams in
from all sides
and in the openness
the searching heart will oblige

This very place we are in—wherever we are—is none other than Tara's emerald sky palace. It is not "up there." It is not "out there." It is just exactly here, now: the light of consciousness that shines in from every perspective in our immediate apprehension (and beyond)—in *nirmanakaya* (gross body), *sambogakaya* (subtle body), *dhrmakaya* (transcendent body), and *svavaikakaya* (integral body) appearances. This light of consciousness is Tara's dwelling place. Here in this space of all-pervading awareness, the heart that searches out compassion, that looks for Tara's face, will definitely find her. The true searching heart will definitely encounter Tara on the spot. There is certainty. There is no doubt. There is recognition of the definitive meaning of the deity's mandalic palace.

the three jewels
adorn your heart
as peace beyond suffering
you make your mark
with your eyes of moon and sun
in your celestial home
there's room for everyone

And the last stanza … "the three jewels / adorn your heart / as peace beyond suffering / you make your mark." Buddha, dharma, sangha. I, thou / we, it. The within, the between, the among, the around. These faces of the integral spirit. These faces of Tara. These aspects, indeed, of your very self, your own mind, inseparable from Tara, adorn your heart. This whole display of appearance–emptiness–appearance, of sacred space, wear them as the jewels that they are within your heart. That is the core teaching of compassionate wisdom. "As peace beyond suffering / you make your mark."

To inquire, what is peace beyond suffering? Of samsara, nirvana inseparable? Milarepa sings "Samsara is not deported to somewhere else; nirvana is not imported from somewhere else" (L. Palden and A. Goldfield, personal communications of Milarepa's song of realization, Sukhasiddhi retreat, 2009). So this is the sound–emptiness–sound echo of that understanding, of that teaching, of that awareness. "With your eyes of moon and sun / in your celestial home / there's room for everyone." So in the traditional depictions of Tara she literally has the eyes of moon and sun and she contains literally night and day; she includes and transcends this world.

Tara is none other than the great Mother of all Buddhas. She is right here in this world. We don't have to go anywhere else to find her. The Buddha of this Earth is none other than Tara's body, Tara's dwelling place, Tara's palace. And in Tara's celestial palace, there is room for everyone. Without a single one left out, including you and me. All sentient beings are in her care.

No sentient being is beyond her embrace: Whether you are anonymous or infamous. Whether you are burdened by debt or buoyed by capital. Whether you are living alone or living in partnership. Whether you are enjoying work, suffering through your work, suffering from lack of work, or enjoying not working. Whether you recognize yourself in all of these guises or many of them or just a select few. In our coming and going, no matter what hardships we have grappled with on this Earth, the divine Mother, Lady Tara, is an inexhaustible source of refuge.

And that is perhaps the essence of our faith. We experience the direct realization that in actuality, we are not beyond love. What's more, we are, in fact, the ground of that pure love. Tara is not beyond us. In truth, she is who we are in our essential nature. The three perspectives of I, I-thou, and it, none other than the three jewels in Buddhism of Buddha, Sangha, Dharma, are adornments, or facets, of that basic truth.

In this way, my nighttime dream of Eva, an expression of the spiritual psyche (Pearson & Marlo, 2021), figures *dreaming soul* and *touching grace.* Here, dreaming demonstrates and transmits Tara's union of form and emptiness expressed variously through sight as "appearance–emptiness–appearance," through sound as "sound–emptiness–sound" and through thought as the "clarity–emptiness–thought" of co-dreaming (Haq & Masih, 2018), through nested dreams, dreaming's reach, and the simulcast of dreams. In this way, honoring the mystery of the soul, the grace of dreaming, in learning from living, is realized as none other than the dreaming of Grace, as Tara.

Dreaming Tara

Eva: Thank you, Willow. I'm curious what feelings are residual in the wake of reading, not just the dream, but also the sound that is there in the emptiness for you?

Willow: Tara's right here in all ways. She is and isn't you and me—and everywhere and everything and everyone. To look for her is to see her appear.

Eva: Returning to the opening nighttime dream, what is the feeling that was arising for you with dream Eva's departure? It seemed to me that there was concern about her departure.

Willow: There was. It's a concern about people being able to contact your expression of love beyond your disappearance and, by extension, our expression of love through this book beyond our disappearance. It is a sense of how I'm wanting to share this book, to let the pages be a vessel for what can be opened through community, expression, dialogue, exchange, communion, collaboration. That this work is meant to be shared, not to be on a shelf somewhere. There's a wish for this book to be a living work.

Eva: Yes. And the departure at 7 o'clock feels like a complete and full exit, which is what it is to be mortal. That at a certain unknown time, we will exit. And yet, as you express—which is really beautiful—the essence, the spirit, is always present and will remain.

Willow: This dream dimension helps me understand something about faith that is organized in various forms of religion, of different religious traditions, as something that people can connect to life after life, generation after generation, person after person, form after form. And that continuity is the importance of lineage: something transcends not only the individual but also a time and place, linking collectives across time and place. I think there's a wish in the dream that the grace of dreaming, the emotional truth of dreams, might participate in a living lineage of honoring the dream and dreaming the dream forward.

Eva: And that this work on the emotional truth of dreams is about a soul lineage, a spirit lineage, beyond blood lines.

Willow: Absolutely.

Eva: This is especially salient given that neither of us have biological children and that biological motherhood is just one form of lineage. Our contribution is in another form, of soul lineage.

Willow: Yes.

Eva: There are multiple streams of soul lineage that we're weaving into this book, that will exist beyond our exit, beyond our departure.

Willow: Yes. Part of the inspiration for writing this book is to facilitate transmission, a soul lineage transmission that, hopefully, can inspire others to also apprentice their dreams as an act of grace. To apprentice dreams as a form of learning from them and also, reciprocally, making an offering to their dreams. To learn from the dream image and to make an offering in turn, to ask what does the dream image want or need from me?

Notes

1 See S. Bloch (2024).
2 Dreaming this Buddhist deity, "Tara's Promise" can be received as a contemporary song of realization in the Tibetan Buddhist tradition of the doha. For traditional songs of realization, see Brunnhölzl (2021, 2019) and T. Heruka (2016).
3 Hear the song, "Tara's Promise" at www.lionessroars.org/music/redboat. You can also hear "Tara's Promise" on streaming and downloadable music services such as iTunes, Spotify, Pandora, Deezer, and Amazon Music, under artists "The Watermoons" (Willow Pearson and Eric Ramstad).
4 This lowercase iteration of "tara" is written here, as I penned the lyrics, recognizing tara in her immanent guise. Then in the further chapter text, written as initial capped, "Tara," I am recognizing Tara in her transcendent guise. In her true nature, she is both immanent and transcendent at once.

References

Adyashanti. (2025, December 2). The Natural Movement of Life #adyashanti #spiritualawakening #opengatesangha #tao [Video]. YouTube. https://www.youtube.com/shorts/FK_y1byMlUo

Bloch, S. (2024). Music as dreaming. In K. Cohen & L. Daws (Eds.), *Primary process impacts and dreaming the undreamable object in the work of Michael Eigen: Becoming the welcoming object*. Routledge.

Brunnhölzl, K. (2019). *Luminous melodies: Essential dohas of Indian Mahamudra*. Wisdom Publications.

Brunnhölzl, K. (2021). *Milarepa's Kungfu: Mahamudra in his songs of realization*. Wisdom Publications.

Haq, S., & Masih, S. (2018). Waiting in the dark. In M. H. Williams & M. B. Acreche (Eds.), *Counterdreamers: Analysts reading themselves* (pp. 81–90). The Harris Meltzer Trust, Karnac Books.

Heruka, T. (2016). *The hundred thousand songs of Milarepa: A new translation* (C. Stagg, Trans. under the guidance of D. Ponlop Rinpoche). Shambhala.

Marlo, H. (2022). Experiencing the spiritual psyche: Reflections on synchronicity-informed psychotherapy. *Jung Journal: Culture & Psyche*, *16*(4), 44–69, https://doi.org/10.1080/19342039.2022.2125770

Pearson, W. (2021). Caesuras of dreaming: Being and becoming, thinking and imagining. In W. Pearson & H. Marlo (Eds.), *The spiritual psyche: Mysticism, intersubjectivity, and psychoanalysis* (pp. 180–201). Routledge.

Pearson, W., & Marlo, H. (Eds.). (2021). *The spiritual psyche: Mysticism, intersubjectivity, and psychoanalysis*. Routledge.

Polit Dillon, M. (2024). *Highly Sensitive Dreamers: The Art of Dreaming About Clients* (Order No. 31761001) [Doctoral dissertation, California Institute of Integral Studies]. ProQuest Dissertations & Theses Global. https://ciis.idm.oclc.org/login?url=https://www.proquest.com/dissertations-theses/highly-sensitive-dreamers-art-dreaming-about/docview/3145940584/se-2

Whyte, D. (2012). *Pilgram*. Many Rivers Press.

AFTERWORD

Sing the Dream that Wakes You Up

The ground and goal of this book is to invite all of us, authors and readers, into esteemed regard for and participation in our own direct experience of dreaming and dreams. The practice we are transmitting in the creation of this text is that of *singing the dreams that wake you up.*

In the process of honoring and waking up to (not only from) our dreams, the method we have entered is one of deep attention to the emotional truth contained within and emanating from the appearances and the confluences of waking and nighttime dream images, ever nested as they are.

It could be said that our method is one of "nonduality-through-multiplicity," in the sense that initial dream resonances welcome an opening into the doubleness of those initial resonances. In turn, these welcome the multiplicity of those dual dream resonances, in a playful, contemplative wonderment of what this guiding dream–truth–drive[1] discloses, questions, furthers, and opens in the process.

Our threefold injunction to "sing the dream that wakes you up; see [and feel] into and through the dream; rest in and as the dream" (see Pearson, 2014), captures the essence of this "nonduality-through-multiplicity." To "see into and through the dream" is to simultaneously look *through* the lens of the dream, adopting its view, to feel its heartfelt sense and, at once, to look *through* the dream, to extend beyond the dream, to be present to the lucidity, the dynamic movement, the changeability of the dream and its dissolution.[2] In this way, to be open to the dream is like looking through a stained-glass window, appreciating all of its detailed shape and mosaic color, while remaining cognizant of its fundamental clear light. For instance, to engage "nonduality-through-multiplicity" begins, in the afterward of the *Teacher and their teachings* dream, in Chapter 9, with an opening to the doubleness of the diamond heart and the kaleidoscope heart, which fosters multiple new dream discoveries.

DOI: 10.4324/9781003591863-15

Another way to open into this "nonduality-through-multiplicity" is through the doubleness of Freud's *dream navel* and the *dream umbilicus* that was touched upon in Chapter 5, "Others: Learning from Multiple Selves." Right within the specificity of the never-before and never-again dream image that coalesces as the dream navel, there unfurls the dream umbilicus, a taproot to the unbounded cosmos. For instance, just as Eva surrenders her backpack (a dream navel, a tethering to specificity), in Chapter 6, "Surrender: Learning from Illness," this resting of the searching self that the backpack can symbolize is the very opening into no-self that illness ushers in (a dream umbilicus, a portal to infinity).

Touching the Essence of Our Humanity: Nonduality-Through-Multiplicity

To further illustrate this dance of "nonduality-through-multiplicity" that follows the scent of emotional truth, here is a nighttime dream that visited Willow in the process of writing this afterword, on September 18, 2024.

> *There is an elder Buddhist master in robes who enters the room, practicing. He is a wise and revered elder—an Asian male teacher with white hair. I continue to write, feeling I should both be acknowledging him in the room and also that I should continue writing, for which I feel both a sense of rightness and a twinge of "Is this okay? Shouldn't I be acknowledging him?" while realizing that I am actually acknowledging him in my continuation of writing. He gleefully and ardently says "Buddhidharma!" as one word. I feel his passion and also his separation from me and my separation from him. Moved, I begin to wash his hair, which is (now) course black. Perhaps he is another?*
>
> *And perhaps he is the same being? Slowly pouring water a bit at a time on his dry hair, the water takes time to absorb; a dirty yellow color begins to stream from his head. He hasn't washed in a long while. I am touched by his humanity and mine, meeting.*
>
> *Another ordained Buddhist teacher, an American woman, lights a candle amid her sangha and it sputters in smoke. Does the flame catch?*

I am unclear, in the dream recall, the next afternoon, which part of the dream came first and which part of the dream followed the other part?

In the afterward, now two days following the nighttime dream's appearance, I am quite focused on the Buddhist master's expression, "Buddhidharma!" in the sense that he does not say *Bodhidharma* (a historical Buddhist master) and he does not say Buddhadharma (a term for the teachings of Buddhism). To me, *Buddhidharma* is like an intimate nickname; and the name itself, together with its squealed exclamation in the dream, is an ambassador of emotional truth. The name is a deeply intimate resonance. And yet, at the very same time, there is a heartfelt sense of separation in the dream. This is the doubleness I am awake to. Holding these simultaneous truths alongside of one another, the dream opens further still … The washing of his hair is notable in that I touch him with my own intimate gesture. In a sense, I offer my own realization born of direct contact. Even so, the water is both running off his hair and also slowly being absorbed. (A place to rest in and, as the dream, a dream navel presents itself.) My touch is felt and also not. Where does the runoff water go? (A dream umbilicus unfurls.)

Similarly, in the afterward, the emotional resonance of the dream directs my attention to the dream question, "Does the flame catch?" For what echoes in the dream chambers of sound–emptiness–sound is not a response of yes *or* no, but a response of yes *and* no and an advance of the importance and relevance *and* the nonimportance and irrelevance of the question itself. These echoes call forth the emotional truth of the open-ended question that includes moment-to-moment revelations, expanding beyond any single response.

The dream appearance is felt into, the emptiness of the dream is touched, and the lucidity of the dream is realized-and-released. The clarity–emptiness–thought of the dream rests just as it is, even as it opens further still. This psychotherapeutic and spiritual practice is rooted in emotional truth.

Mutuality: The Interwoven Tapestry of Shared Dreaming

Our commitment to shared dreamwork, particularly through the intimate practice of dream dialogues, transcends a mere exchange of interpretations. The relationship itself emerges not only as a conduit for understanding, but also as a third body, one that over time, through our devoted nourishment, feels, breathes, imagines, and dreams all on its own. The insights that arise are not solely derived from the content of the dreams or the individual experiences of the dreamer, but rather from the dynamic interplay between us, the resonance of our perspectives, and the shared reveries of our intrapsychic lives. Dream dialogues are not a supplementary activity, an addendum to our personal dream journeys; rather, the act of sharing, of witnessing, and being witnessed in the vulnerable space of our dreams, honors and profoundly supports the deepening of our individual souls and the soul of our friendship.

As I receive Willow's dream about the Buddhist master, I am struck by how, at first, he embodies wisdom outside the self or separate from the self. Through the tender act of washing his hair, Willow begins to merge with wisdom in such an intimate way, no boundary remaining between self and other. This inherent mutuality, where giving and receiving intertwine, reveals the ultimate interconnectedness that lies beneath perceived differences. This principle is illuminated in Chapter 9, "Devotion: Learning from Nondual Love" and Chapter 10, "Departure: Learning from Goodbye." Even within the seemingly asymmetrical dynamics of teacher/student and guide/patient, an underlying current of mutual learning and growth persists. While acknowledging the necessary roles and boundaries that define these relationships, we recognize and honor the reciprocal influence and the shared humanity that bind us. As relational psychotherapists, we believe that our deepest psychological explorations are invariably shaped and catalyzed by our interactions with a trusted other. The soul, when witnessed in this way, discovers its own true nature, its timeless wisdom.

Nothing Is Other: The Democratic Landscape of the Psyche

As foregrounded in our introduction, and as expressed through Chapter 5, "Others: Learning from Multiple Selves," our understanding of "nonduality-through-multiplicity" takes a distinct turn toward the recognition and active cultivation of psychic democracy. This perspective challenges the ingrained tendency to categorize and separate, to establish rigid boundaries between "self" and "other," both within our own psyches and in our external interactions. Instead, we propose a more fluid and interconnected reality, where the myriad voices, aspects, and experiences within us—our multiple selves—are not seen as alien or oppositional, but as integral parts of a larger, unified whole. Similarly, our interactions with others are viewed, not as encounters with fundamentally separate entities, but as engagements with different expressions of a shared human and more-than-human experience.

The practice of psychic democracy involves actively listening to and acknowledging these diverse inner voices, fostering internal dialogue and, ultimately, integration. This internal inclusivity then naturally extends outward, shaping how we relate to the world and to others. By dismantling the illusion of a fixed and separate "other," we open ourselves to deeper empathy and compassion. This approach to nonduality recognizes the inherent multiplicity within unity, celebrating the richness and complexity that arises from the interplay of diverse perspectives, both internal and external.

Thresholds: Navigating the Liminal Spaces of Transformation

The recurring motif of the threshold throughout our work—appearing in Chapter 9, "Devotion: Learning from Nondual Love," Chapter 10, "Departure: Learning from Goodbye," Chapter 11, "Burial: Learning from Death," and Chapter 12, "Ascension: Learning from Divinity"—underscores the profound significance of liminality in the process of psychological and spiritual transformation. Thresholds are the in-between spaces, the transitional zones where the familiar dissolves and the potential for something new emerges. They are characterized by a sense of ambiguity, uncertainty, and heightened awareness, as we stand on the precipice of change, no longer fully in one state and not yet fully in another.

Whether it is the ultimate threshold of death, the initiation into motherhood or fatherhood, the sudden loss of a loved one or some part of one's identity, these liminal moments hold immense power as they force us to confront our attachments, our fears, and our assumptions about reality. By consciously engaging with these thresholds in our dreams and in our waking lives, we cultivate a greater capacity for navigating change, staying present with uncertainty, and allowing for the emergence of new possibilities. The wisdom found in these transitional spaces often lies in surrender to the unknown and trust in the inherent unfolding of life.

Nested Dreams: The Labyrinthine Depths of Consciousness

The phenomenon of nested dreams—explored in Chapter 2, "Watch: Learning from Time," Chapter 7, "Wanting Out: Learning from Cats—Bardo and the Shoji Screen," Chapter 8, "Circle Game: Learning from Cats—Chief and His Exercise Wheel," Chapter 9, "Devotion: Learning from Nondual Love," and Chapter 10, "Departure: Learning from Goodbye"—reveals the intricate and multilayered nature of our consciousness. These dreams-within-dreams suggest that our inner world is not a linear or singular narrative, but rather a labyrinth of interconnected realities. One dream can contain another, which in turn might hold yet another. We begin to experience how sleeping and waking dreams seamlessly interpenetrate. We can learn to awaken to how symbolic representations are constantly interacting. These nested structures challenge our ordinary waking perception of reality and invite us to consider the possibility of multiple levels of awareness operating simultaneously. They can evoke questions—and insights—into the nature of time, spiritual revelation, and the very fabric of our subjective experience.

Dream Mandalas: Mapping the Psyche's Unfolding Wholeness

Our exploration of dream mandalas takes the concept of nested dreams a step further, revealing how these layered experiences can coalesce into interconnected concentric circles. The mandala, as a symbol of wholeness and integration, beautifully illustrates the psyche's inherent drive toward unity. As nested dreams unfold and interact, they often gravitate toward certain patterns, reflecting a central point of integration and radiating outward into interconnected pathways.

These dream mandalas can be understood as psychic maps, charting the timeless presence of the dream within the flow of waking time. They represent the unfolding of inner landscapes, where different aspects of the self and different layers of experience find their place within a unified structure. By attending to the patterns and symbols within these dream mandalas, we gain access to deeper levels of understanding about our inner dynamics, our relationships, and our place within the larger cosmos. They offer a visual representation of the interconnectedness of all things and the inherent wholeness that underlies our seemingly fragmented experiences.

Drawing Together the Threads: Reflecting on the Journey and Looking Ahead

In weaving together these threads of mutuality, the dissolution of otherness, the potent liminality of thresholds, the intricate architecture of nested dreams, and the unifying symbolism of dream mandalas, we begin to envision a holistic understanding of the human psyche and its profound interconnectedness. Our exploration reveals that the boundaries we often perceive—between self and other, waking and dreaming, individual and collective—are far more permeable and fluid than we might initially assume. Through the intimate practice of dream dialogues, we discover the living wisdom of the dreamscape as it emerges and dances. A new third body is born from this relational process: the dreambody itself.

By embracing the multiplicity within ourselves, we move toward a more inclusive and compassionate understanding of the human and more-than-human experience. The liminal spaces of transition, the worlds within worlds of nested dreams, and the unifying patterns of dream mandalas all point toward an underlying wholeness—a psychic landscape where time and space intertwine and where the emotional truth of our dreams unfolds within the context of our lived realities. Ultimately, this journey into the depths of our shared and individual dreamscapes illuminates the inherent interconnectedness of all things, inviting us to embrace the richness and complexity of our inner and outer worlds with greater reverence and awe. May this deeper immersion into the nondual heart of our shared dreamscape continue to illuminate the path toward wholeness, fostering a profound recognition that in the tapestry of being, truly, nothing is other.

Notes

1 See Grotstein (2000) for a formulation of a "truth drive," evolved from Bion's work.

2 See Charles (2004, pp. 43–44) for a wonderful description of Grotstein's transcendent position, which creatively and generatively draws from and "beyond the dichotomy of [Klien's] paranoid-schizoid and depressive positions." Our method of learning from dream dialogues can be accurately described as a method of living Grotstein's transcendent position, which might be helpfully termed the transcendent/immanent position to account for what Grotstein names as the "two arms of O"—at once an impersonal (transcendent) and personal (immanent) embrace. See Grotstein (2000 pp. 300–304) for his brief description and clinical examples of the transcendent position. See Grotstein (2007, pp. 121–134) for a further description of the transcendent position. Also, for reference, see Grotstein (1996). Lastly, see Pearson Trimbach (2023) for a description of the orchestration of psychological positions and developmental levels.

References

Charles, M. (2004). *Learning from experience: Guidebook for clinicians*. The Analytic Press.

Grotstein, J. (1996). Bion's "transformation in 'O'" and the concept of the transcendent position. *Melanie Klein & Object Relations*, *14*(2), 109–141. https://archive.internationalpsychoanalysis.net/2015/05/11/bions-transformation-in-o-and-the-concept-of-the-transcendent-position/

Grotstein, J. (2000). *Who is the dreamer who dreams the dream?* Routledge.

Grotstein, J. (2007). *A beam of intense darkness: Wilfred Bion's legacy to psychoanalysis*. Routledge.

Pearson, W. (2014). Dreaming integral. *Journal of Integral Theory and Practice*, *9*(2), 162–168.

Pearson Trimbach, W. (2023). Psyche's score: Music of the integral psychodynamic sphere and its orbits. *Integral Review*, *18*(1). https://integral-review.org/current_issue/vol-18-no-1-september-2023/

INDEX

Notes: *Italics* indicates figures in the text and page numbers followed by "n" refer to end notes.